M000189803

ZUZA ZAK

SLAVIC KITCHEN
ALCHEMY

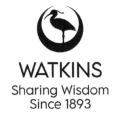

WATKINS
Sharing Wisdom
Since 1893

Slavic Kitchen Alchemy
Zuza Zak

First published in the UK and USA
in 2023 by Watkins, an imprint of
Watkins Media Limited
Unit 11, Shepperton House,
83–93 Shepperton Road
London N1 3DF

enquiries@watkinspublishing.com

Design and typography copyright
© Watkins Media Limited 2023
Text and photography copyright
© Zuza Zak 2023
Cover illustrations copyright
© Shutterstock 2023
Internal illustrations copyright
© Kira Konoshenko & Shutterstock 2023

The right of Zuza Zak to be identified as
the Author of this text has been asserted
in accordance with the Copyright, Designs
and Patents Act of 1988.

All rights reserved. No part of this book
may be reproduced in any form or by any
electronic or mechanical means, including
information storage and retrieval systems,
without permission in writing from the
publisher, except by a reviewer who may
quote brief passages in a review.

Publisher: Fiona Robertson
Project Editor: Brittany Willis
Copyeditor: Sophie Elletson
Head of Design: Karen Smith
Cover Designer: Alice Coleman
Production: Uzma Taj

Commissioned Artwork: Kira Konoshenko

A CIP record for this book is available from
the British Library

ISBN: 978-1-78678-672-2 (Hardback)
ISBN: 978-1-78678-794-1 (eBook)

10 9 8 7 6 5 4 3 2 1

Printed in China

Publisher's note:
While every care has been taken in compiling
the recipes for this book, Watkins Media
Limited, or any other persons who have been
involved in working on this publication,
cannot accept responsibility for any errors
or omissions, inadvertent or not, that may
be found in the recipes or text, nor for
any problems that may arise as a result of
preparing one of these recipes. If you are
pregnant or breastfeeding or have any special
dietary requirements or medical conditions, it
is advisable to consult a medical professional
before following any of the recipes contained
in this book.

Unless otherwise stated:
Use medium fruit and vegetables
Use medium (US large) organic or free-
range eggs
Use fresh herbs, spices and chillies
Americans can use ordinary granulated
sugar when caster sugar is specified
Do not mix metric, imperial and
US cup measurements: 1 tsp = 5ml,
1 tbsp = 15ml, 1 cup = 240ml

www.watkinspublishing.com

FSC
MIX
Paper from
responsible sources
FSC® C104723

ZUZA ZAK

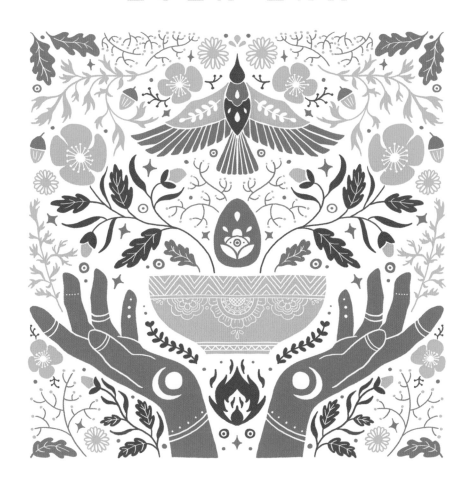

SLAVIC KITCHEN
ALCHEMY

NOURISHING HERBAL REMEDIES,
MAGICAL RECIPES & FOLK WISDOM

DEDICATION:

For my Babcia Ziuta, whose spirit forever remains in the fields and forests, and for my family, for whom I strive to grow

CONTENTS

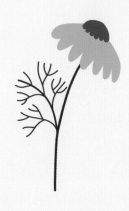

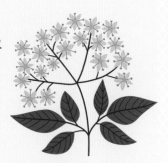

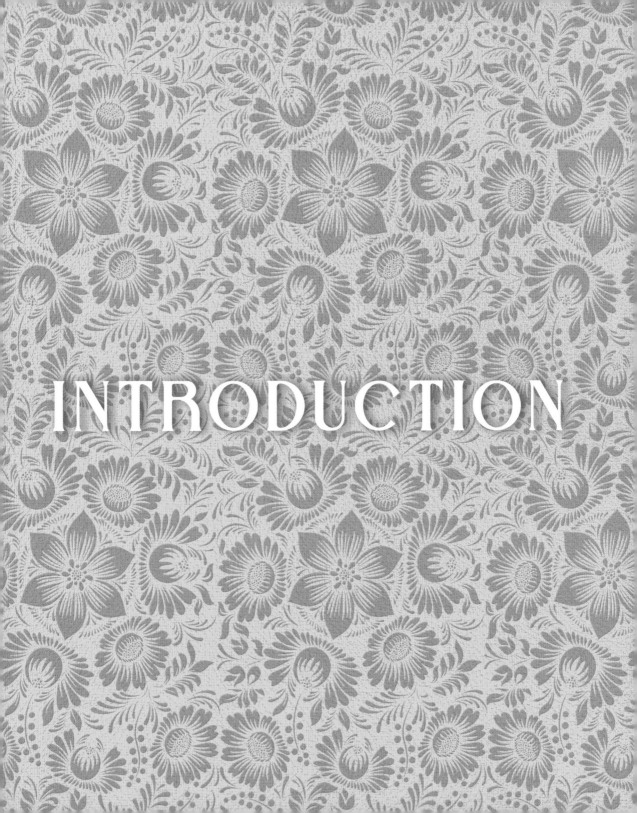

INTRODUCTION

Remembering the Old Ways

The old ways are calling us back, gently yet convincingly. Too long have we been disconnected from the earth and its rhythms, our ancestors and ourselves. This book is my journey of remembering and reconnecting with the nourishing rhythms of life through the lens of Slavic lore: ancient mythology, sacred plants and kitchen tables past. I believe that we have much to learn from this forgotten world. This is a book infused with old Slavic wisdom, passed on to me both by my own grandmothers and other wise women I have met along the way.

There's no need to sugar-coat the past – the old Slavs lived extremely difficult lives. I don't want to go back in time, to where I work the fields from sunrise to sundown, while rearing 12 children with no access to modern medicine. Yet in our speedy quest for ease, we are in danger of losing some fundamental life wisdom. Therefore, we are now faced with a choice: what do we choose to take with us into the future and what do we choose to let go?

I choose to preserve the ancient wisdom of my ancestors, to use the gifts we have been given on this earth to nourish myself and my family and to live in balance with the rhythms of nature. It has taken me a long time to get here, for while those instincts have always resided in me, I was too busy and distracted to embrace them. Then I realized that my goal to be more in touch with that part of myself didn't require some huge change of lifestyle; it's all about the small changes and the everyday connections. I focus on simplicity because this shouldn't be a difficult journey. Everything in this book can be made in a home kitchen without any special equipment or fuss. The point is that by exploring the old ways, we can make our own modern lives feel more connected, more vital.

I believe that many of us are already turning toward the past (or thinking about doing so) in order to understand how we should

move forward. The world around us, the climate, the politics, are tricky to navigate, so perhaps we should be looking to a simpler time when we were more in tune with the earth's rhythms. Perhaps we can even bear to give up some of our modern-day conveniences for the good of the whole and a slower, more conscious pace of life ... This is what I am attempting in my own life.

This book is a treasure trove of old ways, rather than a manual – like an old notebook given to you by your grandmother. I don't advocate any kind of extremity in the way we approach the rituals within these pages. They are simply things to make your life gentler, sweeter and more joyful. Take what you will.

While alchemy might sound otherworldly, we use the elements to transform the properties of things all the time. Cooking uses fire to transform our ingredients, and even breathing is alchemy. For me, alchemy also holds a deeper meaning, because I am committed to transforming myself internally. Therefore, reading books that help me do that is also alchemy. In this book, you will find alchemy on many different levels.

We still say that the kitchen is the heart of a home. It is where we cook and nourish ourselves, but it is often also a meeting place, somewhere to congregate and connect. Historically, Slavic homes started with a kitchen, to house the all-important stove that would feed the household and provide warmth. People therefore cooked, ate, slept and did everything of importance in the kitchen.

The Slavic World

At the time of writing this book, the Slavic world is in turmoil. Many of us are sad, angry and very raw from the war in Ukraine. Folk traditions have nothing to do with imperialism and war; they are about life and healing. This book celebrates the positive aspects of Slavic folk traditions and wisdom, as used through the generations.

Slavs are the largest ethno-linguistic group in Europe, traditionally living in Poland, Ukraine, Russia, Slovenia, Slovakia, Czechia, Belarus, Croatia, Serbia, Bosnia, Montenegro, Macedonia and Bulgaria, although many are, of course, all over the world now. Sadly, At times I feel that there are negative connotations to calling yourself Slavic in the Western world, as if it means you have certain narrow views and possibly nationalistic tendencies. Or that you want to live in the past and worship the old gods. Yet I believe that in the future, tradition and modernity can and will peacefully co-exist.

To truly appreciate the wisdom and beauty of the old Slavic ways, we must get to know more about Slavic folklore and traditions. Only then can we let go of any preconceptions. Slavs are spread across many Eastern European countries and therefore Slavic cultures, languages, customs and cuisines vary. Yet there are also many common threads running from one country to the next, which I will be exploring and celebrating in this book. I am Polish, so you may notice a bias towards Polish folk traditions and stories, as this is what I have been raised with. I speak the language fluently, therefore I know the folk names of some of the plants, which sometimes refer to their qualities. For example, yarrow in Polish is *krwawnik*, a word that comes from "blood" in Polish – *krew* – and the plant was often used to stop bleeding. Because the Slavic languages developed from proto-Slavic, they have the same roots, which means there are many similarities. I use my knowledge of Polish as an opening into the wider Slavic world.

My Babcias

I think of *Slavic Kitchen Alchemy* as my late Babcia (grandma) Ziuta's book. My Babcia had a hard life, full of toil, yet she was a powerful woman. I'm always amazed by her stories from World War

II when she was just a teenager. Twice she was in a situation where the Nazis were threatening to destroy her life. Both times she asked them to let her and her husband go and they did (her brother ended up in a labour camp, starved to the bone, though he did make it out alive). I don't think she even knew how she managed to make her own will triumph in these impossible situations. The first time, she was rounded up when she went to run an errand in Warsaw. She told me that she went up to a soldier, showed him that she had milk for her baby, told him that she needed to go and feed him and he allowed her to escape. Perhaps the fact that she was a young fair-haired girl with blue eyes helped. The second time, soldiers were going from house to house, taking the men away to labour camps. My grandfather was being taken away and my grandma fell on her knees and begged them to let him go. They left him. Perhaps she was lucky to find soldiers who were not convinced of the correctness of their actions. What I do know is that my grandmother had a way of appealing to humanity, of believing that there was some good in everybody, that made people act better in her presence. While she would never have described herself as powerful, I would say that's a great power to have.

My Babcia Ziuta came from the Mazovian countryside before they swapped their land for a modern apartment in a Communist block. She was a cook by profession and at home. She went to church every morning and had the most unwavering faith in God, or *Bozia*, as she lovingly called God, making this omnipotent power feel like a member of the family. In the kitchen, she would cook for her huge extended family and many of the neighbours, too. She never measured anything (even when making her multi-tiered, elaborately decorated cakes) and never wrote anything down. She had an encyclopaedic knowledge of plants and their uses – not their Latin names, of course, but their country names. One of my biggest regrets is that I didn't write down all the information she passed on

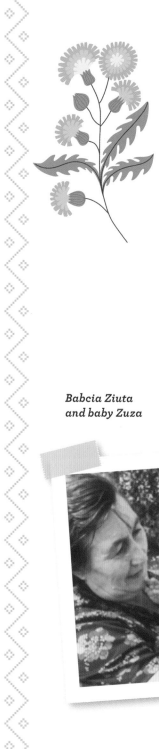

to me when she was alive and I still remembered it all. How I wish that as a teenager, instead of journaling my tumultuous emotions, I'd jotted down all the gold-dust knowledge that a country walk with my Babcia Ziuta would produce. But wisdom is for the old, and you can't blame a child for not doing research for books they will write in their adulthood. I've managed to remember a lot and while this may seem farfetched to some, I feel that my grandma has been guiding me in my research – from the books I have read, to the people I have spoken to, to the articles and manuals that have magically appeared on my doorstep. This book has been a journey of remembering and rediscovery.

My Babcia Halinka was originally from Lithuania. She had been expatriated to Olsztyn in the northeast of Poland after World War II and finally settled in Warsaw later in life. She had studied law, was extremely political and opinionated and wrote all the time. She wrote a whole trunkful of diaries throughout her life, as her mother had done before her. Traditionally, diaries and documents go on the fire when a person dies – a letting go of all they were in this life. For this reason, she never passed on a notebook of favourite remedies and recipes, yet I did find a lot of the clippings she had collected through the years. Many of them are herbal remedies and little-known regional Polish recipes. I cut them out and stuck them in a notebook myself. I invite you to treat this book as a notebook too, so please make notes in the margins and attach cut-outs of things that interest you.

*Babcia Ziuta
and baby Zuza*

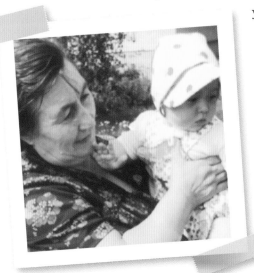

Religions and Folklore

Slavic folklore and Christianity have gone hand in hand for hundreds of years. Through my own family, I understand that faith has brought immense comfort to people in times of grief; it has brought warmth and hope when there was none, and it has kept people going when it seemed impossible to do so. However, when you know Slavic culture from the inside, you realize that there is something hiding underneath the Christian faith, something that makes that faith uniquely Slavic. Rather like Shinto co-exists with Buddhism in Japan to create a uniquely Japanese version of Buddhism, the old ways are still alive within Catholicism in Poland, which makes that religion experientially different to Catholicism in Italy, for example.

The main Slavic gods survived by morphing into Christian figures; for example, Weles took on the role of Saint Nicholas in Ukraine, while the ancient God of Thunder, Perun, morphed into Saint Elijah. Sadly, some of the smaller deities were demonized in the process. This focus on good versus evil in medieval Christianity meant that pagan "enemies" were needed to fit in with the story that the Church was correct, good and there to protect us from evil.

In this book, I aim to go deeper in search of the Slavic wisdom that lies beyond the limitations of the Church and the fear that has been sown throughout the years. I seek to find the old ways and beliefs that have been preserved within Slavic homes. Many of the old Slavic traditions ran so deep that they couldn't be forgotten and ended up being absorbed into the Church, such as the tradition of Easter egg decorating – *pisanki*. It's difficult to believe now that our most important Polish Easter tradition of taking painted eggs to Church in a beautifully decorated basket with other food to get them blessed was, in fact, banned in the first two centuries of Christianity. Eggs were associated with pagan magic. There was even a type of healing in which you rolled an egg around your body. Decorating eggs was

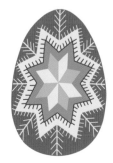

practised exclusively by women (I imagine because they are seen as life givers) and involved various superstitions, which would have added an air of danger to the innocent act.

Ancient Slavic beliefs are even more elusive than their practices. They were passed down through word of mouth, and as such, Slavic folklore didn't exist as a whole in the minds of the people; the beliefs were fragmented and changed from one area to the next. Nevertheless, they must have been strongly ingrained, for we still feel their presence now in our collective imagination, even though Christianity has been the dominant religion for over a thousand years. It is this Slavic folklore, with its old gods and goddesses, magical animals and spirits, that I love to piece together and explore, uncovering that which has been hidden. However, it's equally important to note that many herbs are associated with the saints or the Holy Mother, and when the old ways are used it is often in conjunction with the Christian faith. Due to the belief that herbs are even more potent when they are blessed by a priest, there are days in the year when herbs are ritually blessed – our Lady of Herbs, 15 August, is the main one in Poland. Many folk healers also believe that their power is directly given by God and that even though they are using old methods, they are undeniably doing God's work.

A Journey of Rediscovery – Folk Healing and Magic

Slavic magic would generally have been practised by people who are in some way enlightened into the magical arts. They could perform spells and incantations, or teach them to people who would then perform them as instructed. It was something that most people participated in at some point in their lives, whether for good or evil. The old word for witch – *wiedźma* or *wiedźmin* – comes from the (Polish) word *wiedzieć*, meaning "to know" (and I imagine it's similar in other Slavic

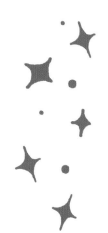

languages). These people living on the outskirts of villages were both feared and respected (rather like the old gods) for their knowledge and power, and were visited often by the villagers, who did not have access to the medical care we have these days. Historically, in Russia, it was men who were most often accused of witchcraft rather than women. In Siberia, there is a history of shamanism that is still practised today. *Szeptuchy* – the women whisperers – of the Polish folk tradition, can still sometimes be found in remote villages, although they are not as common as they were in the past.

Folk healing is not the same thing as magic. Folk healing is for everyday use – we use plants and nature to help our bodies regain their balance. It's generally done on a daily basis in one way or another, because it pertains to daily worries, such as a cold or indigestion, or to basic improvements that we would like to see, such as shiny hair or a glowing complexion. Even in modern times, when I go to my homeland, I see people using elements of folk healing that have become traditions in their family or that have been passed on through word of mouth to help with a certain ailment. It is folk healing that we focus on in this book, not magic. However, there is clearly an overlap. My Babcia Ziuta was an extremely devout Catholic and using plants to heal was never considered to be witchcraft by either her or those around her. She was simply practised in the old ways – folk healing. Nevertheless, I have been told that my grandma would, when it was needed, very rarely and in private, perform strange rituals with incantations – one involved licking eyelids and spitting in every corner of the room. When I was a baby, she once performed a ritual on me involving the throwing of salt, to try and get rid of colic. Rituals such as this were probably to get rid of some kind of perceived evil and protect the recipient. Personally, I do not do spells or incantations; however, like many Slavic people, I love a bit of gentle divination, through tarot, tea leaves, wreaths or even walnuts! In terms of manifesting what I want, I make my wishes very clear, often writing them down or saying them out loud, like a simple prayer. I believe that in the modern world we have come to pigeonhole things in unnecessary ways, which sometimes leads us to separate ourselves from things that could be beneficial to us.

In Eastern Europe, plant medicine has been studied alongside allopathic medicine, even during Communist times. There is no concept of "alternative medicine" because the two worlds are not mutually exclusive. After all, most medical drugs are originally derived from plants, so there is no need for such a disconnect between the two. Thanks to research, there are certain plants that are no longer used in folk medicine, such as ragwort. This common plant, which looks rather similar to St John's Wort (and is also known as St James' Wort) used to be added to Polish *nalewki* – vodka medicines – as well as made into infusions to treat cramps. I expect that it must have been effective, otherwise people wouldn't have used it. However, it is now known to damage the liver, therefore we avoid it. Our family friend Marta, who grew up in a Polish village, told us how when her father was struck by lightning that came in through the fireplace, her mother acted very quickly and found super-human strength (adrenaline) to pick him up and shake him. This probably saved his life, as the electricity was grounded through her body. However, before the ambulance came, and against her mother's wishes, the villagers took him away and buried him in the ground, covering him in mud to "ground" him. That probably didn't help, as it only made him cold and wet.

I believe that folk medicine can complement modern medicine, not replace it. Therefore, as I repeat throughout the book, don't use any of these folk remedies to replace prescribed medication. While they are powerful, this is not an exact science – a plant has many compounds that may affect your body in various ways. Moreover, you won't know the exact quantities you would need, and if you consume too much of something, you could be in danger of suffering from ill side effects.

WHAT'S IN A NAME?

In folk wisdom plants go by many names. Even in the Polish language, I have come across plants that will have up to 30 folk names, and then there's all the other Slavic languages. Therefore, while I might mention a Slavic (Polish) name, for example when the folk name is relevant to the use of the plant, I have decided to stick to the English and Latin names, for ease and safety.

Gods, goddesses and mythical beings are also known by many names; however, there are usually similarities between them, so that they are recognizable from one Slavic language to the next. As I am Polish, I often use the name I am most familiar with or the name from the country where the cult of that mythical being is strongest.

Wisdom and Superstition

Separating wisdom from superstition is like removing the grain from the chaff. I have spent many an hour trying to understand the difference between the two and I have finally come to the conclusion that the main difference is in how it makes you feel. If you feel fear, a foreboding, a grasping for control, then it's probably superstition. If, on the other hand, something makes you feel elevated and inspired, then that's wisdom at work. In my research, I found that many Slavic folk stories were filled with fear and foreboding in order to teach people harsh lessons. I certainly do not want to be passing on fears, as that's the opposite of what this book is about. The stories in this book, even if a little dark at times, will hopefully elevate and enrich you.

The Slavs were, on the whole, incredibly superstitious people. In the past, I have struggled with the superstitions ingrained in my own psyche, believing that they were an intrinsic part of my Slavic identity. Eventually, I realized that I needed to move toward the light in my life, rather than hold on to the ancestral fears, which have been passed down the generations.

You can understand why superstition is a huge part of folk culture when you take a moment to imagine the harsh reality of village life throughout the ages. Times when your life and the lives of your loved ones were dependent on external factors, such as weather conditions, diseases, enemy attacks and a religion that was highly politicized and imposed on top of the original pagan beliefs. Superstition gives you the illusion of control, which provided a sense of comfort. Ironically, I've found that it's only when I let go and stop trying to enforce control that things work out like they're supposed to. Nevertheless, that's easy to say when living a privileged First World life. Imagine you're living in a village, and the villages around you are suffering from some terrible illness. What you do to protect yourselves will draw upon every tool available to you, be it magic, superstition or wisdom. In Poland, string was sometimes used to encircle a village in order to protect it. I expect that people felt safe within that magical circle and that belief would, in turn, give them at least some form of protection.

With all the superstition and the fragmentation within the Slavic belief system, it has been too easy for critics to write off folk wisdom as being unenlightened. Yet, I believe that with discernment, we can gain much practical wisdom from holistic and multifaceted folk culture. In his ethnographic book of 1891, Marian Udziela wrote about the numerology prevalent in folk beliefs. He highlighted the numbers three, seven, nine, 13 and 27 as being the most vital in folk medicine and applied them in a myriad of ways that sometimes did not make sense to outsiders. Perhaps these numbers could be seen as mindless superstition, yet Udziela understood the origin of this folk numerology to be from the "Jewish-Arabic Kabala" tradition. When I talk about Slavic culture, therefore, I am talking about it from a wider perspective than people might have these days. We must remember that Slavic folklore is not some hermetic, secret society. Folk culture by nature is open and embracing. There's an element of magic to it, but it's also deeply practical. It's based as much on faith as it is on trial and error.

How To Use This Book

This book isn't meant to be followed with religious fervour or to replace anything you are already doing to take care of yourself. It's meant to be an enjoyable way of exploring the old Slavic ways and finding additions to your daily rituals that will benefit your mental and physical health.

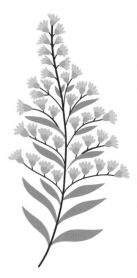

I would encourage you to begin reading from the season that you are currently in to get a sense of what feels inspiring. Start there. Take a pen and make notes in the margins, circle things, crease the pages and amend the recipes to your liking. Generally, I invite you to make this book your own, like your own grandma's notebook that you can pass on to younger generations in time, if you wish.

When you have an ailment, look upon this book as your old, wise Slavic aunt, who wants to help you with the treatments that her mother or grandmother passed on to her. This may be pleasant, like a herbal tea or a shot of sweet spirits, or it may not be, like onion syrup (see page 144). In any case, I believe it's worth a try. I have only included the things that work for me. The ancient Slavs tended to view illness as an outside being that entered the body. They would try various things to remove the harmful entity, yet once it was there, it wasn't easy. Therefore, they knew full well that health needed to be preserved from the start. Their whole system was based on using nature to maintain good health.

This book is about nourishing our body and souls into a state of balance and wellbeing. If you are on medications, then please seek advice from your doctor before taking any herbs to make sure that they won't adversely affect your treatment (herbs are very powerful). If you are advised to avoid the internal usage of certain herbs, you can still feel connected to the seasons and the earth through a topical recipe or a cream. Sometimes, tiny changes in your routine can bring surprisingly positive results.

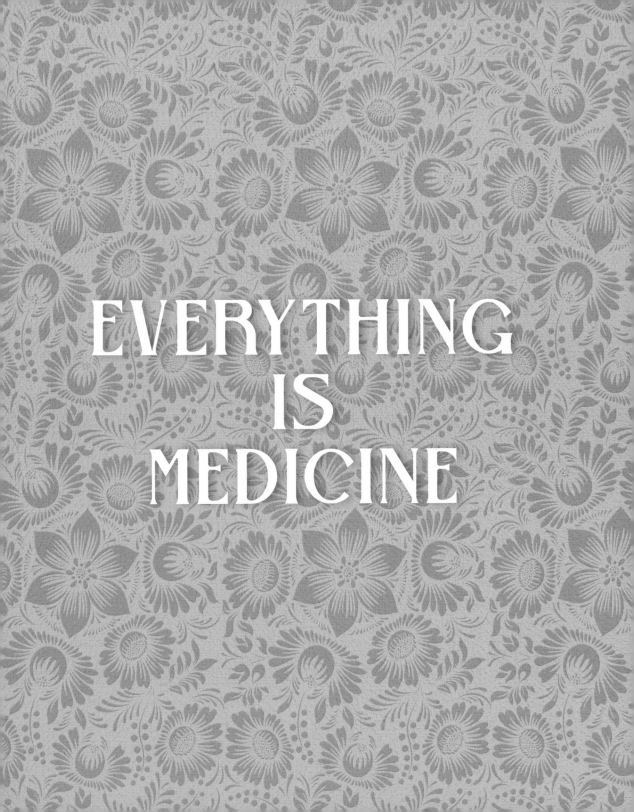

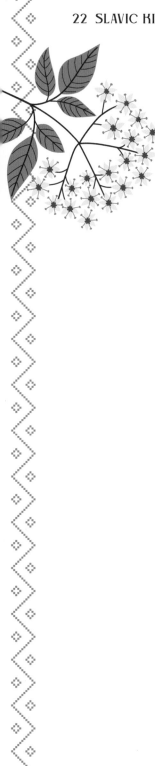

Natural Ways to Nourish and Heal

There is a saying that "everything is medicine" and I believe that there is some truth to it. We can choose to view everything as being useful and, in many ways, this book is about finding out how to use the plants around us to nourish and heal. However, each person is unique, therefore what is helpful to one individual isn't necessarily helpful to the next. While one person might benefit from adding some seasonal Slavic rituals to their daily routines, for another person that could feel unnatural and they might gain wisdom from reading stories, analysing themselves and applying folk wisdom to their lives instead. While one person might need some time working with their hands in meditative craft, another might need to focus on connecting to nature. Personally, I have a few daily practices that never change – for example, my daily yoga practice – and in addition I have seasonal rituals, which connect me to the earth and vary according to her and my rhythms. These changeable practices are where I connect to my Slavic roots. They are also dependent on my mood, the time I have and my needs at that moment.

Lake swimming is something that I have done since my childhood in Poland and has stayed with me to this day. I consider it to be a magical blessing in my life, especially since a swimming lake came into existence so close to where I live shortly after I moved in! I do this throughout the warmer months. Similarly, foraging is something that I have been doing since I was young. In Communist Poland, it was a way of supplementing our diets, but it was seen as a hobby rather than a necessity. It's a way to be in nature and to connect to the seasons. There are various folk "rules" to picking mushrooms, such as, "Don't keep your knife out, because the mushrooms will hide away" and "Don't talk or you'll frighten the mushrooms," which, if you abide, can make the whole experience akin to Japanese-style forest bathing.

In the spring, I will always find time to pick nettles for stews and wild greens for salads. In the summer, I will pick local berries and sorrel from the fields for soup, and in the autumn, there will be acorn cookies and rosehip tea. I have now added foraging for tree bark to my winter rituals, thanks to the work of a Polish couple who call themselves *Chwastożercy* – the weed eaters. Learning how to forage in winter was a revelation to me. It's important to nourish ourselves in the harsher months of the year and one of the simplest ways of doing this is eating wild foods that grow in our local area, for I believe that they contain the antidote to anything in the atmosphere that could be harming us. I prepare *nalewki* – Polish vodka medicines – whenever the mood takes me, in order to preserve plants that are seasonal and just for the fun of it. I find that they are one of the most pleasant medicines to take. Half a shot a day as needed is ideal for me, and it lifts the spirits too!

I also turn to certain remedies in a more cyclical way and as needed. For example, during my monthly cycle, I know that a yarrow infusion will help soothe my stomach (see page 146). When I have a cough and/or cold, I will always eat a piece of rye bread and garlic (see page 171), do inhalations (see page 143) and drink infusions made with plantain and/or other herbs (see page 142).

From time to time, I will take on a more complicated endeavour, such as spending a cosy evening making some seasonal decorations around the kitchen table or performing a special ritual in private.

The main thing I have learned about myself in my 43 years on this planet is that I need balance. This involves using what the earth provides at the right time – therefore being seasonal but without being militant about it. I make a habit of listening to the earth and my body. It does not mean that everything I eat is organic, but I will not eat an animal that has been kept in unhappy squalor or drink milk that has been produced at the expense of a cow's wellbeing. It is my intention to support systems that support the earth and our future

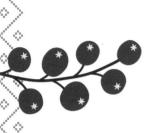

on it. This is a responsibility that we have as consumers and it's time to take this seriously, because this is a way that we can heal not only our bodies but also our planet – a way that's available to every single one of us. In fact, this book takes us away from being consumers for a moment, because most of the remedies are free or very cheap. As my physiotherapist, Magda's, Slavic grandmother used to say to her: "God plants around your house everything you need", meaning that there will be things growing near where you live that can help with whatever health issues you might be prone to. Take a look around.

THE LANGUAGE OF PLANTS

Isn't it interesting that plants that are often seen as noxious weeds can have so many benefits hidden within them? Perhaps those most beneficial plants are also the most resilient ones that know how to survive, and the time has come to tap into their wisdom.

Slavic Kitchen Alchemy focuses on plants that have been used for the past few hundred years in Central–Eastern Europe. They are not all native, as there have been trade routes since antiquity and, with them, an exchange of knowledge in all its forms. In our globalized society, there shouldn't be a problem finding these plants wherever in the world you reside.

Growing plants ourselves can be a brilliant way to connect with nature and to know exactly what we are picking. What we grow depends on our situation. I began growing my own food when I was living in London, in containers with limited access to water. I found that some common plants are next to impossible to grow (chamomile, lovage), while others were surprisingly simple (sunflowers, mint). I also found that some plants just miraculously appeared in the containers, such as wild rocket.

Not every plant that our ancestors used worked in the way it was intended to. Of course, after many years of personal experience and that of her ancestors who passed the knowledge down, my Babcia basically knew what worked and what didn't. She also had wonderful common sense, which stood her well, as superstition was prone to being mixed up with actual wisdom. In this book, while commenting on superstitious beliefs for fun, I have decided to stick to what I find works, using modern research to my benefit. For example, the old remedy of hot milk with butter and honey for a cold, however comforting and lovely, has now been proved to have some adverse effects (we should avoid mucus-causing dairy foods when we have a cold), while the rye bread with garlic that was served with the milk is spot on and I still use this cold remedy today.

These are the various methods of nourishing and healing that we will explore in this book:

FORAGING

Foraging is the most natural way to connect to the earth and something that humans have always done. The act itself feels life-affirming and the goodness that we take from those plants surpasses anything we can buy in a shop – and it's also completely free. However, there is always a risk with foraging, which is multiplied, and thus can be frightening, for beginners.

With certain plants and mushrooms, you have to be extra careful. If a plant has an extremely poisonous lookalike, then I prefer to leave it alone. For example, I tend to stay away from cow parsley as it looks way too similar to hemlock (and giant hogweed, some say) to be worth picking for me. I used to happily pick and eat parasol mushrooms in Poland, knowing how they differ from the poisonous white toadstool and verifying each one with my uncle Kazik, who I consider to be an expert. However, then I spoke to a family friend, Greg, who is a doctor that used to work on a toxicology ward in Poland. He said every year he saw at least a handful of people who had made a deadly mistake with that particular mushroom, so I have decided that the risk, however small, is simply not worth it.

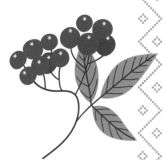

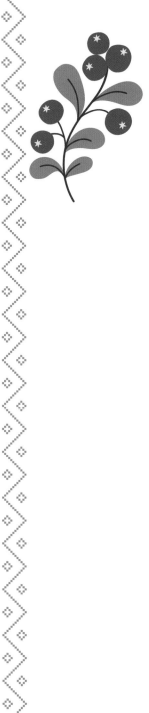

Here are some foraging rules that I swear by:

Rule one: know exactly what you are picking. Don't rely on just one source, unless it's a human expert who is absolutely sure, otherwise you need to cross-reference. Almost every flower or mushroom has a toxic counterpart that it could be mistaken for. Recognizing plants has become much easier these days with apps that immediately tell you exactly what you are looking at. However, with ease comes complacency; therefore, I must urge you to always seek a second opinion. Use an app and a book, for example, or better yet, an app and an expert. I use the Picture This app for plants, but I even double check plants that I'm 100 per cent sure of and catalogue them on my app. If there is any doubt at all, discard it, because it's just not worth the risk. Ideally, we would all have a foraging mentor – someone who knows exactly what they are doing and can pass their knowledge on. When I go to Poland, these mentors are everywhere, as everyone seems to have huge amounts of knowledge of at least some part of the subject that they are prepared to share.

Rule two: only take a small amount. You should not be taking more than a fifth of what you find in any one place. We need to be respectful of the earth, because we are not here just to take, take, take. It's a two-way relationship, so we should be conscious of not disrupting the habitat, and, if we are taking leaves, then we should leave the roots and/or bulbs where they are. If, like with burdock, we are taking some roots, then make sure you leave others where they are, unless you need to remove this plant entirely (for example, if it's on farmland).

Rule three: pick quality. Find a spot away from any roads and other disturbances and pick the youngest, greenest, freshest leaves you find.

Rule four: ask for permission. This rule is dependent on where you are foraging. In the UK and Poland where I forage, the land is public property, but in some countries, a lot of land is owned by someone.

Rule five: leave all rare species alone. I believe that all the plants I forage and that I talk about in this book are in abundance. However, this might not be the case in other parts of the world. Please double check before you forage.

The ancient Slavs thanked the trees when they picked from them, and I tend to preserve this tradition of gratitude when foraging.

PLANTING AND HARVESTING

Ideally, we would plant a seed a few days after the new moon, once the thinnest of crescents appears in the sky, so that it grows with the moon. We would harvest around a full moon, as that's the natural end of a cycle. While I don't always follow these old ways, I do enjoy the process even more when I do.

Herbs are known to have the strongest potency when freshly picked, therefore I tend to pick them just before use. In addition, Slavic folk wisdom dictates that picking herbs just before they flower also adds to their effectiveness. So, if at all possible, when you see buds appearing it's a clear sign to start picking and using. In terms of the time of day, many believe that herbs, greens and flowers should be picked once the dew has dried, but before midday. There even used to be rules about which direction to pick the plants from, so that they catch the sun correctly as you pick them, or what the weather should be on the day you harvest. This is a step too far for me, however. Once I have picked the herbs, I give them a quick, gentle rinse under cold running water, then shake them a little to dry them and leave in a sieve until I need them.

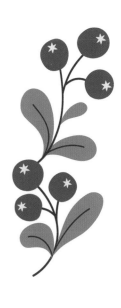

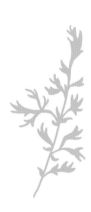

✦ **Drying:** Before drying plants, we need to rinse them under running water and allow them to air-dry in a sieve. If they are still a little moist, then you can gently pat them with a clean dish towel. Most plants will be fine being dried in a warm oven on its lowest setting (around 40–50°C/100–120°F) for 3–4 hours on a baking sheet lined with greaseproof/wax paper. Make sure that they are well spaced out.

RECIPES

Cooking is alchemy. For me, cooking and recipes hold the deepest significance, and this is why I have been working with food for much of my life (I have written three cookbooks). Recipes talk to us of history and of the people that came before us, therefore through cooking we are communing with nature and with our ancestors. In this way, all recipes are magical. However, in this book, I have gathered the most magical ones, the most wild and special, all with a Slavic history, which I hope will allow you to fully experience the earth's seasons, wild nature and the Slavic ways.

✦ **A note on recipe titles:** the recipe titles are meant as a guide. Each plant has a myriad of health benefits, so I have chosen the one that they are best known for and what I personally use them for.

INFUSIONS/TEAS

One of the simplest and most universal ways to use herbs is in an infusion. They are so simple that to a cookbook author like myself, they seem to be non-recipes. Yet infusions are powerful. For example, one that I learned about from my mama is yarrow. Once when I had a mild upset tummy that refused to go away within a couple of days, drinking this simple, tasty infusion soothed it immediately. I just couldn't believe that I'd waited for two days! On the other hand, when I once drunk some of Mum's digestive herbal mix, I gave myself a horrible stomach upset. I recommend you test as many infusions in this book as possible, then continue to use the ones that work for you.

When a plant is in season, I do fresh infusions, which is an ideal way to look after our health and practise self-care. If an infusion is working well for you, then make sure to dry some flowers/leaves for the future, for when you might need their properties but they are not in season.

DECOCTIONS

A decoction is somewhat like an infusion, but it involves boiling the plant matter in water, in order to get the goodness out. This can be beneficial when a plant has hard leaves or we are using the bark of a tree.

NALEWKI

We aren't used to thinking of alcohol as "nourishing" or helpful in the West, yet a *nalewka* is like a tincture (works on same principal) with an element of pleasure added in. I somewhat feared that including vodka medicine in this book would either put people off or make them think they can drink a lot of it, neither of which is the result I'm aiming for. Yet to leave *nalewki* out would feel like a crime to Slavic folk medicine.

Neither of my Babcias drank alcohol, yet a shot of *nalewka* was taken at times, with health in mind. In etymological terms, a *nalewka* is simply something that is poured. Physically, it is a vodka with the health-giving properties of the herbs that it was made with. In terms of folk customs, it is an almost daily medicine. My Babcia Halinka favoured *nalewka* made from aronia/chokeberries (see page 101), while my Babcia Ziuta always had some *orzechówka* on hand (see page 55) for the stomach. A *nalewka* is made with spirytus (90 per cent alcohol) in Poland, which is then watered down to a percentage closer to vodka. However, as spirytus is not available everywhere, we shall stick to vodka in this book.

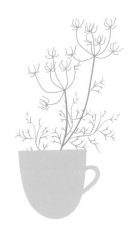

SYRUPS

Syrups or cordials are thick, sweet preparations that are meant to be drunk in small doses. More often than not they are meant for children. However, from time to time, I do a course of one myself; for example, elderberry syrup when summer turns to autumn (see page 103) and I need an extra immunity boost, but I want to avoid the alcohol in a vodka medicine. Syrups are usually based on sugar these days, but I think it's safe to assume that the old Slavs would have used honey for these kinds of preparations, as they used honey both to sweeten and heal. Therefore, I give both options.

VINEGAR

Apple cider vinegar (see page 148) is the ancient vinegar that has once again gained popularity because of its health-giving properties. The ancient Slavs used it not only in cooking, but to disinfect wounds, in cleaning and in beauty products.

OILS

This book is for everyone to use at home; therefore, it doesn't include any practices that are tricky and/or require any special equipment. All the oils in this book are infused oils, although sometimes I may suggest using a drop or two of essential oil, which you can buy from a healthfood store or online.

The carrier oils that I use are the ones that are traditional to a Slavic kitchen, but you can replace my suggestion of sunflower and flaxseed oil with sweet almond oil or another carrier oil. Flaxseed oil is very beneficial to the skin; however, it also has quite a strong smell, so I would maximize both the amount of herbs used and the infusing time when using this oil.

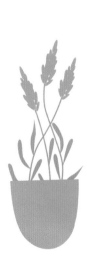

INHALATIONS

This is one of my favourite ways to cleanse both the skin and lungs. I do inhalations year-round, often just grabbing a few leaves from the geranium that we have as a house plant in the kitchen for a quick five-minute facial spa. When my daughters have a cold, I put them to sleep, then boil some water and pour it into a bowl in their room with either a spring of mint or a few drops of peppermint oil. This helps them to breathe in their sleep, which is of course the main objective, because that's when our bodies heal the fastest. Before I go to bed, I will often refresh the bowl.

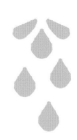

FOLK TALES

"Stories are medicine"
Clarissa Pinkola Estés, *Women Who Run with the Wolves*

Folk tales are stories that have been passed down orally through the ages in order to teach us vital life lessons, thereby nourishing our spirits. Each storyteller adds something new to the tale or tells it slightly differently to the last. In this way, folk tales evolve and become a fascinating reflection of the ever-changing culture of a place and its people. As the current storyteller, I am not hugely concerned with recounting the folk tale precisely; I recognize the essence of the story, then retell it in my own words.

The folk tales in this book are all from various Slavic cultures. Stories are older than national boundaries, therefore it's very possible that some may have been recorded as originating from one country, while also being present in others. I implore you to focus on the medicine inside the story. What is it teaching us? What feelings does it bring up for you? Let's think about how we can apply this to our own lives.

FOLK ARTS AND CRAFTS

Art does not need to be lofty and well marketed to be of value. While I am interested in modern art, folk art is like medicine to me. It is based on the natural human need to connect to something beautiful, and greater than ourselves. It is what makes us human. The Wieliczka Salt Mine in the south of Poland is a wondrous underground world created by miners who simply felt the need to create something of beauty out of the resource available to them: salt. Their art raised them out of their ordinary existence and into the realm of the spiritual – true divine inspiration.

I have always been a huge fan of folk arts and crafts from the whole world over, although, of course, I will delve more into Slavic folk arts and crafts in this book.

While I hugely appreciate the medicine we can find in folk arts and crafts, I am no expert in this field; therefore, I have consulted with my friend Karolina Merska (author of *Making Mobiles: Create Beautiful Polish Pajaki From Natural Materials*), who works as a cultural anthropologist in this field.

COSMETICS

Natural cosmetics are something I have enjoyed dabbling in since an early age. Don't we all make perfumes from flowers as children? In this play, there is a natural inclination to make our own natural beauty products. This interest in beautifying ourselves is an old one, and the Slavs had their own preferred herbs and food items that they used for this purpose. Some were more universal, such as using the sacred linden tree and apples – apple cider vinegar, mainly – while others were more personal beauty secrets that I have learned from word of mouth. I have shared my favourite ones in this book, and I hope that you add your own in the margins (with a view to passing it on to future generations). For example, you can make an oat bundle that is perfect for cleansing and exfoliating the skin (see page 41), or you can use a burdock and nettle rinse for strong, shiny hair (see page 96). The beauty products in this book are always straightforward to make, but if you use normal water rather than distilled water, please make sure you discard the product after three days and make another batch.

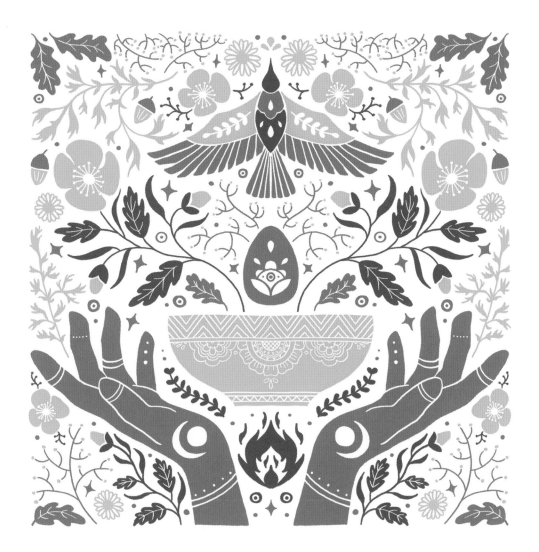

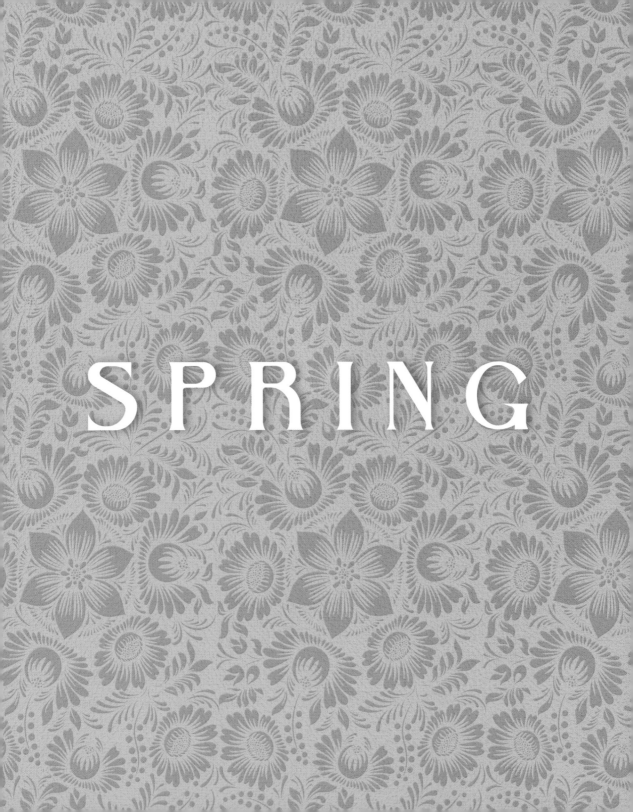

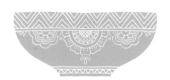

After the harsh months of winter, spring is a time to be celebrated in the Slavic lands with magical rituals that hark back to pagan times. But first, there's the fasting of Lent and ritual spring cleaning, including burning herbs to clean the space of any illnesses that winter may have left behind.

In Poland, Lithuania and Slovakia, the spring equinox is celebrated with the "drowning" of Marzanna – a Slavic goddess who symbolizes the harshness of winter (also known as Morena and Morana and sometimes even Śmierć, which literally translates as "death"). An effigy made of straw and dressed in rags is danced around, dipped in puddles and paraded around the entire village in order to collect any illnesses and worries, before being ceremonially burned with herbs and thrown in the river at dusk. This is a goodbye to winter and a celebration of the rebirth of the earth. Folk superstition dictates that you don't look back at Marzanna once she's in the water.

Saying goodbye to Marzanna marks the end of winter. Some say that it was the young, lively Dziewanna who then came to create the beauty and life of spring (though she is better known as the hunter goddess). This is also symbolized by the *Nowe Latko* – New Summer – ritual a few days later, when a large pine branch adorned with colourful decorations such as eggs and ribbons is carried into the village. An even older ritual was called Wypędzanie Zimy or "chasing away the winter" took place on the first Sunday of May, when a spruce tree would be decorated with colourful ribbons and paper decorations and carried around the village by the children of the house to celebrate the changing of the seasons.

In the Poland of my childhood, Palm Sunday would bring paper and straw flowers wrapped with colourful ribbons - *palmy*. In pre-Christian times, boys and girls would gently whip one another with pussy willow branches to drive out winter illnesses – the pussy willow being a Slavic symbol of health, fertility and strength. What's left of this tradition nowadays is Śmigus Dyngus – Wet Monday – when we pour water over one another. In my youth, I remember being woken up by being squirted with water from a plastic egg. Older boys would often go much further (too far, some might say) and wait at windows with entire buckets of water to pour over unsuspecting girls. However, while being drenched in cold water was a shock, this would always be taken in good spirits in the end, as the common understanding is that the wetter the girl gets, the luckier she will be in the future.

In the spring, we want to reconnect with the earth. Slowly at first, perhaps with some seasonal recipes using foraged ingredients. Then, once we get into May, I would encourage walking barefoot on grass whenever possible. This is something Polish people, and many other Slavs, seem to have ingrained in them. When my mum's city-dweller friends come to visit her in the countryside, they immediately take their shoes off and walk on her lovely lawn. For maximum benefit,

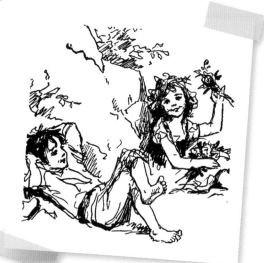

we would do it for 20 minutes a day, but even five minutes is better than nothing.

Spring planting takes place after Zimnej Zośki, as 15 May is known in Poland. Zimna means "cold" and Zośka is the diminutive for Zofia, the saint whose day is 15 May. In folk custom, we also talk about *zimni ogrodnicy* – the "cold gardeners" – any of whom may bring some frost up until mid-May.

Polish folk wisdom also teaches us to look to the cycles of the moon when sowing our plants. Seeds should never be sown on either the full or new moon. We wait until a few days after the new moon, when the crescent is growing, to sow our seeds, so that they grow with the moon. May was the month of Mary, and so many people started foraging at this time, believing the herbs to be at their maximum potency. While some only collected herbs in May, others believed that to have the most healing powers, herbs need to be collected before the day of Saint Jan (John), which falls on 23 June.

When spring meets summer, the countryside celebrates Zielone Świątki – the Green Holiday – which comes at Pentecost in the Christian calendar and marks the end of spring. The most important aspect of this is "greening" the world with newly cut branches of trees, thereby ensuring health and abundance, and protection from lightning. The birch tree is the tree of choice at this time of year, for it is known to bring positive energy. In Poland, calamus was used to sweep the porch. It's a herb that came with the Tartars from the East (hence it's Polish name: *tatarek pospolity*). It grows near the lakes and rivers, and is known to have cleansing, antibacterial properties. In some areas, it's thrown on the floor in a particular pattern, filling the space with a fresh, citrusy fragrance.

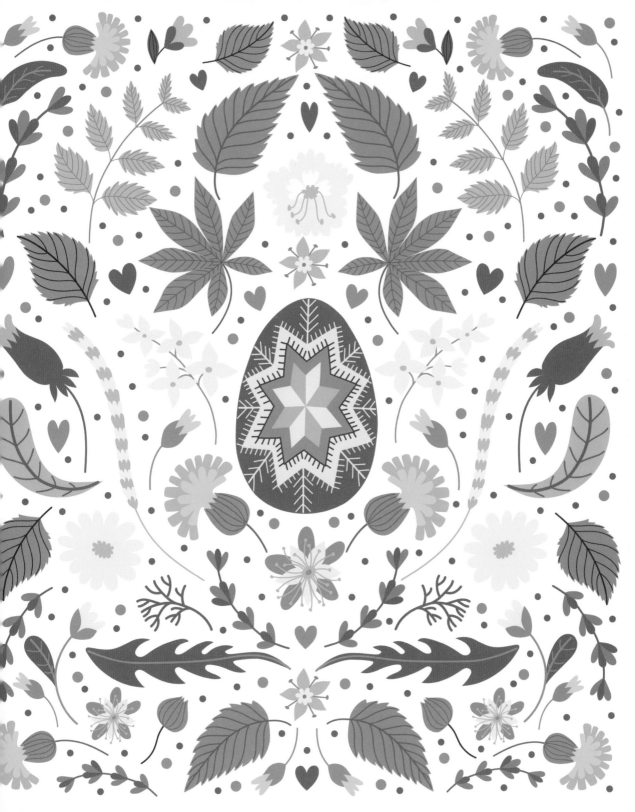

SAGE CLEANING SPRAY for ritual spring cleaning

First things first, in spring we need to clean our homes. Spring cleaning was a vital part of spring preparations in the old Slavic cultures. We do this as early as possible in spring, ideally at the same time as Lenten fasting. Of course, in the modern world, we may be dieting rather than fasting and religion may not come into play at all, yet the rhythms of nature remain the same, and before the new, we must give order to the old and get rid of everything that is no longer serving us. Doing this in the physical world, externally, will then spur the same kinds of changes internally. The two go together.

As my mother will testify, regular cleaning was not my strong point when growing up; other things always took priority. However, as I have matured, I've started to see the benefits of a clean space. Your mind also feels clearer. Therefore, in order to make sure the most important things get organized during spring, this is what I do: on my weekly list of priorities, I add just one area that I would like to clean. It could be a whole room or a part of a room, such as an oven (for an oven I would use this sage spray in conjunction with baking soda) or even just one messy, crowded shelf. Sometimes, it's even a bag or a box. This activity never takes longer than 30 minutes, so that it's possible to slot it into my busy schedule. Sometimes, I even do it with one of my children. In this way, I can clean 12 areas during the three months of spring.

Sage (*Salvia officinalis*) has many uses and one of the traditional ways it was used was to purify. Combined with vinegar and alcohol, it makes a potent, yet natural cleaning spray. Since the olden days, spirytus – Polish alcohol – has been used in Poland for cleaning both things and people. We can use any kind of 80–100 per cent alcohol for this and, ideally, a glass bottle.

Follow the below steps to sterilize glass jars and bottles.

◉ Preheat the oven to 160°C/ 315°F/Gas mark 3.

◉ Wash the jars and lids in hot soapy water, then rinse. Don't fully dry them.

◉ Arrange the jars in a roasting pan and place in the oven for 10 minutes.

◉ Soak the lids in boiling water for a further few minutes.

◉ Allow to dry naturally.

MAKES 1 X 250ml/9fl oz BOTTLE

3 sprigs of sage
50ml/2fl oz/scant ¼ cup distilled water
100ml/3½fl oz/scant ½ cup 80–100
    per cent alcohol
50ml/2fl oz/scant ¼ cup white vinegar
250ml/9fl oz sterilized glass jar
250ml/9fl oz sterilized glass spray
    bottle

◙ Muddle the sage sprigs in a
pestle and mortar until they release
their oils.

◙ Add the distilled water to the
pestle and mortar and keep muddling
for a few more minutes. Pour into a
sterilized glass jar. Add the alcohol
and white vinegar and shake
vigorously.

◙ Allow to infuse for 3 nights, then
strain out the sage and pour into your
spray bottle.

◙ Shake and use to
clean every surface
of your home. Use
within 2 months.

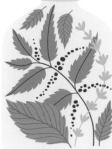

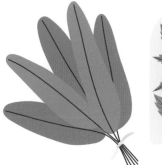

OAT BUNDLE CLEANSER
for gentle exfoliation

As we shed our winter layers and
clean our surroundings, letting go
of everything we no longer need, we
must start thinking about our skin. A
simple yet effective way of exfoliating
and softening the skin is to use an oat
(*Avena sativa*) bundle. I like to have
one for my face and another one for
my body. The amounts below are for
one bundle, which will last for about
five days. If you would like to continue
exfoliating after that time, you should
make another bundle with a clean bit
of cloth. However, I would recommend
giving your skin a rest for about a
week. Use a 30cm (12in) square of
cotton, ideally quite thin.

MAKES 1 BUNDLE

200g/7oz/2 cups rolled oats
1 cotton muslin/cheesecloth, soft dish
    towel or thin cotton napkin
1 elastic band

◙ In a food processor, blitz the oats
to a flour-like consistency.

◙ Place the ground oats on the piece
of cloth, make a bundle to enclose the
oats and tie at the top tightly using an
elastic band to keep it together.

◙ To use the cleanser, wet the
bottom of the bundle and apply to
wet skin in circular motions. Rinse off.

PURIFYING HERB BUNDLE for incense cleansing

Smoke purifies. We can maximize its effect with herbs that have been used since ancient times. Even cattle used to be cleansed with incense to protect them from witchery, because witches love cow's milk!

While there are many herbs that we can use for incense, in bundles we need to use those that burn easily and evenly. All the herbs I suggest here have some kind of cleansing, purifying effect. You can add or remove herbs to your liking, so that your bundle is customized to your needs. Use the top 20cm (8in) of each plant.

Make sure you burn the bundle with everyone out of the house and the windows open. The amounts opposite are for one bundle, for one deep-cleansing session, to be done after spring cleaning.

All the herbs have purifying qualities and are widely available. Mugwort (*Artemisia vulgaris*) has been used in Slavic herbal medicine for thousands of years, but in large quantities it could be toxic, so be careful with young children. It is collected during flowering, near the end of April.

MAKES 1 BUNDLE

2 sprigs of peppermint
(*Mentha piperita*) or
spearmint (*Mentha spicata*)
1 sprig of nettle (*Urtica dioica*)
1 sprig of thyme (*Thymus vulgaris*)
1 sprig of sage (*Salvia officinalis*)
1 sprig of mugwort
(*Artemisia vulgaris*)
20–30cm (8–12in) piece of
natural string

◉ Dry all the plants on a newspaper in a warm but shady spot for about 24 hours.

◉ Bundle them together, making sure they are the same length and snipping where necessary. Tie the bundle snugly with the string. To do this, tie a knot at the bottom, then wind it around three-quarters of the bundle so that only a few leaves stick out the top.

◉ Hang this upside down in a warm, dry place (but out of the sun) for a week or two.

◉ Light the top of the bundle. Walk around every room of your house, placing the bundle in each corner of the room for a couple of seconds.

◉ You can also cleanse yourself at the end of the ritual, by wafting the bundle around your body, from top to toe, for a minute or so.

◉ To finish, press the bundle top down into a heatproof container.

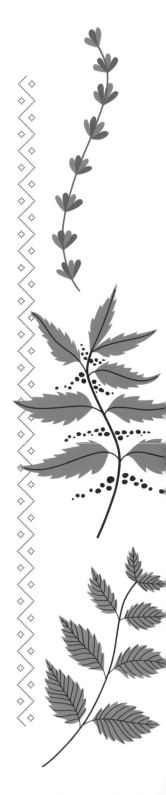

BABKA (PLANTAIN)
for disinfection

Every child in Eastern Europe probably knows that if you fall over and graze your knee, to stop it from bleeding, you put a babka on it. In my generation, at least, this was common knowledge. In England, I've found this plant described as "a troublesome weed". However, the broadleaf plantain (*Plantago major*) has many benefits and could be seen as nature's gift (if a smooth lawn is not your main priority).

First and simplest of all: if you have a cut or a graze that won't stop bleeding, place a babka leaf on it and hold it firmly in place for a minute or so. Teach your children to do the same. This is one of the most useful things to know, as these leaves can be found everywhere. Of course, later, they can go and get it cleaned and seen to at home, but this is an immediate antibacterial compress. It also helps with insect bites in much the same way. I would recommend spitting on the babka first, in order to clean away any dust or dirt.

If the wound is more serious, and you are a while away from receiving any medical help, then you can create the following compress while you wait.

MAKES 1 COMPRESS

10 babka leaves
1 length of gauze dressing
   (about 30cm/12in)
1 large cotton wool square or
   clean cotton muslin/cheesecloth,
   folded to the right size

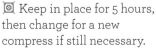 Clean the wound of any visible dirt with warm water.

◉ Wash the babka leaves well, then crush them in a pestle and mortar until they release their juices.

◉ Place the leaves on the cotton wool square/muslin and over the wound. Tie the gauze to keep the compress in place.

◉ Keep in place for 5 hours, then change for a new compress if still necessary.

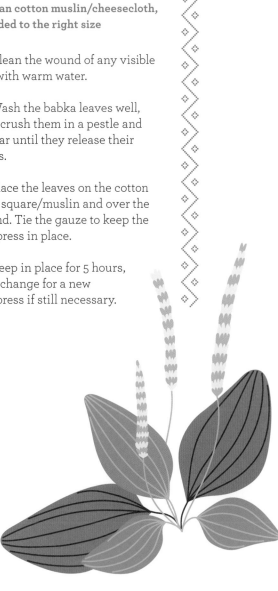

CHAMOMILE BATH DECOCTION for relaxation and optimism

When I told my English friend in passing that I bathe my baby in chamomile, she said it sounded like a very witchy practice.

While chamomile (*Matricaria chamomilla*) is used in many baby products, it's often so diluted that we don't really get the full benefits of the herb. Chamomile is known to have a mildly cleansing, antibacterial effect, and therefore it's perfect for the whole family and especially for babies. Sunny chamomile symbolized happiness and goodness for the ancient Slavs and has so many uses that I advise picking it whenever you get the opportunity (there are many lookalikes, so make sure that you are picking the right thing).

If I don't have any dried chamomile to make an infusion, then I will use ordinary chamomile tea bags. I brew a couple of bags for at least 10 minutes to get a strong potency, then add it to the baby's bath water or use it to clean the baby instead of giving them a bath (it has been scientifically proven that babies should not be bathed every day, though this could be due to the manufactured bath products that cleanse away the natural skin oils). Often, I will join my babies in the chamomile bath because I enjoy its calming properties. If I am menstruating, I will drink a chamomile tea instead. In this case, I would use 60 flowers and an extra cup of water and as soon as the water bubbles, ladle out a cupful, sweeten it with honey and cool slightly before drinking.

Wild chamomile flowers are best if you can pick ones growing away from roads. I remember picking them with my Babcia as we walked along country roads. These roads ran alongside fields, so there wasn't much pollution to worry about.

To dry:
Lay the flowers outside in a shady spot for awhile, before continuing the drying process inside for a further few days.

MAKES 1 DECOCTION

40–50 fresh or dried chamomile flowers
1l/35fl oz/4¼ cups water

◙ Place the chamomile flowers in a large saucepan and cover with the water. Bring to the boil.

◙ Simmer for 10 minutes, then turn the heat off and allow to cool until warm.

◙ Strain and add to a bath.

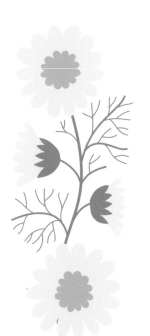

LILAC BODY OIL
for soft skin and improved intuition

Deeply and unapologetically floral, lilac (*Syringa vulgaris*) is one of my favourite smells, as it reminds me of spending time with my Babcia Halinka. There was a lilac bush growing outside her apartment block and we would stop and smell it every time we went past. Even though my Babcia's favourite perfume was rose, it's lilac that I always associate with her. Lilac has a whole host of other skin-toning properties, so it seems a shame to just use it as perfume; therefore, I have created a lightly perfumed oil you can use to moisturize your whole body. Some say that lilac oil even improves your intuition and psychic abilities. I always felt that there was something magical about it!

Notes:
1. *Make sure you first test the oil on a little patch of skin.*
2. *Taking the lilac flowers off the stamens is painstaking work, and since we are not eating it, there is no need to.*

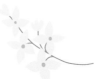

MAKES 1 x 250ml/9fl oz BOTTLE

4 heads of lilac, flowers removed
200ml/7fl oz/scant 1 cup cold-pressed sweet almond oil or sunflower oil
250ml/9fl oz sterilized glass jar
250ml/9fl oz sterilized dark glass bottle, optional

SUNSHINE METHOD

◉ Fill the jar with the lilac flowers (leave the others on the branch until you need them) and pour over the oil. Close the lid and leave in a sunny spot.

◉ After 5 days, strain the flowers out and pour the oil into a dark bottle if you wish. You can keep it at room temperature for 2 months.

SPEEDY METHOD

◉ Fill the jar with the lilac flowers.

◉ Heat the oil until it's very warm but not hot (about 40°C/100°F). You should still be able to keep a finger in the oil.

◉ Pour the oil over the lilac flowers. Close the lid and leave in a sunny spot for 2–3 days.

◉ Strain the flowers out and pour the oil into a dark bottle if you wish. You can keep this oil at room temperature for about 2 months.

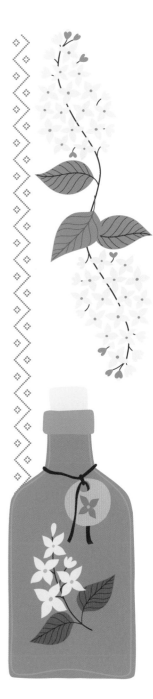

SPIRITS OF NATURE

As a child in Poland, we would often go to stay by a lake. In the evenings, I'd swim out as far as I could into the middle of the water, where the sun had lit it up, so I could swim in magical waters of molten silver without being observed from the shore. This felt like its own realm, an unseen one. I'd pretend I was a *rusałka* – a water spirit. I instinctively felt the rusałki to be otherworldly and ethereal, but also playful and fun.

Rusalky were eventually demonized in Christian times. They were even rumoured to drown men by tickling them to death and other such fantasies. Yet they have been a part of the ancient waters of these lands for far longer than that. In Poland, another word for *rusałki* is *boginki*, which means "goddesses", suggesting that they may have been worshipped long ago. In Serbia, these spirits of nature were called *veela*, often armed with bows and arrows and said to help humans with their knowledge of herbs. One thing that all Slavs agree on is that these beautiful female spirits love to dance and sing.

Zielone Świątki – the Green Holiday – is a Slavic festival associated with these female deities. It usually takes place at the start of June (sometimes it's the end of May), with feasts given in their honour and offerings of bread, eggs and other food left for them by the river. After all, they were the deities of the spring rain, which was necessary for crops, so even if feared, they had to be appeased. Even now, *rusałki* remain a symbol of beauty and grace, adorning themselves with wreaths of wildflowers and herbs. In some countries, such as Serbia and Croatia, it is believed that these wreaths have magical powers.

Mamuny, on the other hand, were said to be vengeful spirits of nature. As they are also female and also reside in forests, rivers and lakes, perhaps the two deities have become confused with one another at some point in time, resulting in the innocent *rusałki* getting a bad reputation. *Mamuny* are said to be the spirits of women who died in childbirth or committed suicide in these places. Their deep unhappiness has made them vengeful and cruel. After the birth of a child, people feared that *mamuny* would swap the baby or torture the new mother. Interestingly, it's St John's Wort that was said to protect the mother from the sadness and torment inflicted by *mamuny*, a herb that is now universally used to treat depression.

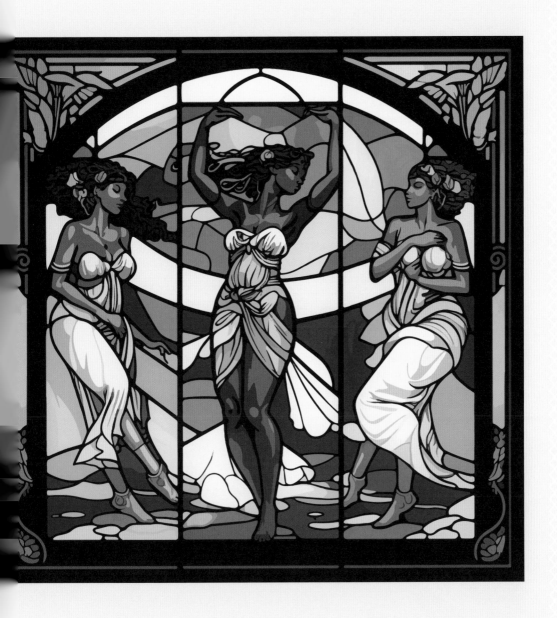

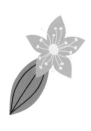

ST JOHN'S WORT NIGHT-TIME BATH for relaxation and a happy glow

St John's Wort (*Hypericum perforatum*) is a powerful herb and has many uses, not only as protection from malevolent deities. I suggest a spring bath in these flowers, as they contain many compounds that are wonderful for the complexion. The flowers can make your skin extra-sensitive; so avoid exposing yourself to strong sunlight straight afterwards. This is why I recommend the St John's Wort bath as a night time ritual. For an extra soothing, calming effect, use a little of the St John's Wort infusion to make yourself a bedtime tea.

Remember to pick flowers that grow away from any roads. Pick the top 20cm (8in) of the plant. We want to use both the leaves and the flowers.

To dry:
Place the sprigs on a newspaper in a well-ventilated spot for an hour or so, to allow any bugs to depart, then tie with the string and hang upside down in a warm, dry place for 3–4 days.

MAKES 2 BATHS

2 sprigs of St John's Wort
20cm (8in) natural string
400ml/14fl oz/1¾ cups warm water
   from a pre-boiled kettle

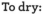 Take half the sprigs out of the bundle and place in a clean jar for a future bath, breaking them up as you do this. Break up the other sprigs and place in a bowl.

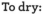 Pour the warm (but not hot) water over the St John's Wort in the bowl, then cover and allow to infuse for 20–30 minutes.

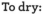 If you would like to make yourself a cup of St John's Wort tea, then take 50ml/2fl oz/scant ¼ cup of this infusion and top up with 100ml/3½fl oz/scant ½ cup hot (not boiling) water and sweeten with honey.

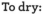 Pour the rest of the St John's Wort infusion into your bath. Pick off the leaves and flowers and place them in your bath too.

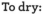 Soak in the bath for 20–30 minutes.

LINDEN BUD INFUSION for a blissful spring afternoon

Wispy, delicate linden blossoms have always seemed to me like fairies floating in the sky. Their fragrance is spring itself – delicate, slightly shy, yet persistent. In Polish, the month of July has been named after the linden tree (*Tilia cordata*), as this is when it fills the countryside with its fragrance and aura. You can find out more about this sacred tree in the Summer chapter (see page 92). For this infusion, we need the early buds of spring. If you find some early-blooming flowers, then feel empowered to pick them too. Linden buds have been proven to have calming, sedative properties. You could also deduce this through their smell, because even taking a deep breath under a linden tree will make you feel calmer and more blissful. The flowers, leaves and bark have been used in folk medicine throughout the ages to that effect.

SERVES 2

2 tablespoons fresh linden buds and flowers (1 tablespoon if dried)
400ml/14fl oz/1²/₃ cups hot water from a pre-boiled kettle
1–2 teaspoons good-quality honey

◉ Place the linden buds and flowers in a teapot and cover with hot (not boiling) water. Close the lid and leave to infuse for about 10 minutes.

◉ Strain into your mugs or a thermos flask and stir in the honey.

HONEY

HORSE CHESTNUT FLOWER BATH to reduce cellulite and relax the body

Many folk practitioners claim that horse chestnut (*Aesculus hippocastanum*) flowers have a strengthening effect on the entire body and reduce things like cellulite and dark shadows under the eyes. Therefore, a bath is the ideal way to make the most of their properties.

When you get in the bath, wet a small face towel with the bath water and place it over your face to make sure that the face and eyes get a relaxing treatment too. As with any foraging, make sure to choose trees that are well away from busy roads.

To dry:
Place the flowers on a baking sheet lined with greaseproof/wax paper and leave to dry slightly before use. Leave them in a well ventilated area for 6-12 hours. If you are saving some for the future, continue drying for a further 12 hours.

MAKES 2 BATHS

40–50 horse chestnut flowers
400ml/14fl oz/1⅔ cups warm water
  from a pre-boiled kettle

◉ Place half the dried flowers in a bowl (the rest can go in a screw-top jar for another time) and pour the warm (but not hot) water over the top. Cover and allow to infuse for 20-30 minutes.

◉ Run yourself a hot bath and pour in the water infused with the chestnut flowers.

◉ Soak in the bath for 20-30 minutes.

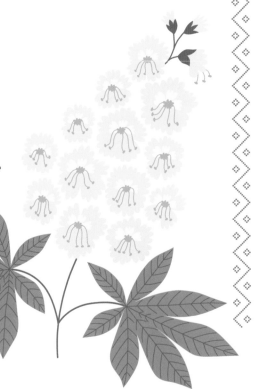

DOCTOR'S DANDELION "HONEY" for strength

We were gifted a jar of treacly, dandelion (*Taraxacum officinale*) "honey" by a Polish friend, Marta, an avid nature lover and forager. This isn't honey, of course, but has the same consistency and sweetness and, reportedly, some great health benefits, including strengthening the liver, stomach and kidneys. It tastes great on top of some yogurt with nuts.

Firstly, we need to distinguish between the common dandelion (*Taraxacum officinale*) we need and the other one (*Taraxacum platycarpum*), as both are equally common. While all dandelions are edible, the dandelion flowers we want for this recipe have their own stem with no leaves on it. In Polish, this plant is called *mniszek lekarski* – the "doctor's dandelion", fittingly. Please check with a good book or guide if you have any doubts as to what you're picking.

Secondly, we need to make sure that we are foraging it from a good source, where the environment and the earth have not been polluted. While this is true of all foraging, the dandelion is particularly sensitive to any kind of pollutants and absorbs everything.

MAKES 1 X 250ml/9fl oz JAR

100g/3½oz dandelion flowers
250ml/9fl oz/1 cup hot water
   from a pre-boiled kettle
250g/9oz golden caster/
   granulated sugar
Juice of ½ lemon
250ml/9fl oz sterilized glass jar

◉ Place the dandelion flowers on a dish towel and leave on a sunny windowsill for about 30–40 minutes, to allow any creatures to depart.

◉ Wash the flowers well under running water, shaking them a little afterwards, then place in a large saucepan and cover with the hot water. Bring to the boil, turn the heat down and simmer for 15 minutes over a low heat.

◉ Take the pan off the heat, cover and leave to infuse for 24 hours.

◉ Strain the flowers out of the liquid and discard.

◉ Add the sugar and lemon juice to the pan and mix well. Simmer for about 90 minutes over a very low heat until it thickens.

◉ Transfer the "honey" to your sterilized jar, close the lid and place upside down until it cools.

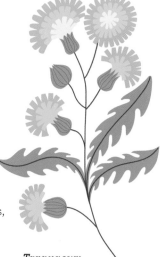

Taraxacum platycarpum

Use *Taraxacum officinale* (flowers on their own stem with no leaves)

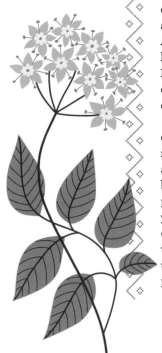

ELDERFLOWER MIODOWNIK CAKE for immunity and the sheer joy of it

I'm a great fan of helping the body in ways that are joyful, and this delicious cake is a wonderful example of that. Why not boost your immunity while eating a beautiful, fragrant cake? Elderflower (*Sambucus nigra*) has been used in natural medicines to help the body's natural responses to various viruses for generations.

This cake is based on the famous *Miodownik* cake (also called *Medovik*) known in various guises all over Slavic lands since the Middle Ages. While honey was used to sweeten cakes in the olden days, when it was used in large amounts, the cake was then called *Medovik* or *Miodownik*, which literally means "honey cake". Here, we are uniting the benefits of honey and elderflower for a delicious immunity boost.

In many East European countries, this cake consists of many wafer-thin layers. I wanted a simpler, quicker version for this book, since not everyone wants to put so much time into a cake, when you can make an equally delicious cake with less effort. This is like the Polish *Miodownik* that I grew up with, with only three layers and plenty of elderflower cream filling.

MAKES 1 CAKE

FOR THE ELDERFLOWER SYRUP
20 elderflower heads
Zest of 1 lemon
200g/7oz caster/granulated sugar
450ml/15½fl oz/1¾ cups of water

FOR THE CAKE
200ml/7fl oz/scant 1 cup good-
   quality honey
150ml/5fl oz/⅔ cup elderflower
   syrup (see above)
200g/7oz butter (salted or unsalted),
   plus extra for greasing
500g/1lb 2oz/3¾ cups plain/
   all-purpose flour, plus more
   for dusting
Large pinch of salt
1 teaspoon bicarbonate of soda/
   baking soda
1 egg, lightly beaten

FOR THE FILLING
800g/1lb 12oz/3½ cups mascarpone
   or cream cheese
2 tablespoons icing/confectioners'
   sugar
1 egg yolk
5 tablespoons elderflower syrup,
   plus extra for brushing

FOR THE TOPPING
Icing/confectioners' sugar
Handful of elderflowers

◙ Preheat the oven to 200°C/
400°F/Gas mark 6 and grease a
20cm (8in) square loose-bottom
cake pan.

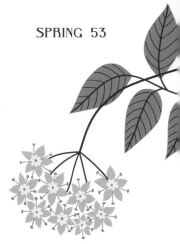

◙ To make the elderflower syrup, gently wash the elderflower heads and place them in a medium pan with the lemon zest and sugar. Cover with the water and bring to the boil, stirring until the sugar dissolves, then turn the heat down and simmer for about 20 minutes, covered. Turn the heat off and allow to cool to room temperature, before straining through a sieve.

◙ To make the cake, pour the honey and elderflower syrup into a small pan and cook over a medium heat for 5–10 minutes, or until it turns a shade darker.

◙ Meanwhile, heat the butter in a frying pan over a medium heat until it turns golden brown (about 7–8 minutes). Turn the heat off.

◙ Gently pour the honey mixture into the browned butter and stir thoroughly to combine. Transfer to a large mixing bowl and allow to cool until it's warm.

◙ Sift the flour, salt and bicarbonate of soda into the bowl with the wet mixture, add the egg and mix well.

◙ While your dough is still warm, tip it onto a lightly floured surface and knead for about 5 minutes until it's very soft. Divide into three equal portions.

◙ Working with one piece at a time, roll out the dough until it's the shape and size of your cake pan, then press it into the pan and bake for 10 minutes, or until browning slightly around the edges.

◙ Turn the cake out onto a wire/ cooling rack. Once your pan has cooled, repeat with the remaining two pieces of dough. Use a knife to even out your edges and break these offcuts into large crumbs.

◙ To make the filling, whisk the mascarpone, icing sugar, egg yolk and elderflower syrup together.

◙ To assemble, brush your base cake layer with 2 tablespoons of elderflower syrup, then spoon on 3 tablespoons of mascarpone filling and spread it evenly over the surface. Repeat with the remaining layers, finishing with a layer of the filling. Sprinkle this final layer with your crumbs.

◙ Chill the cake in the refrigerator overnight (for at least 12 hours) so the moisture soaks the layers. To serve, sprinkle the offcut cake crumbs on top, dust with icing sugar and scatter with more elderflowers.

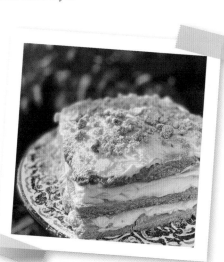

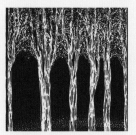

THE HEALTH– GIVING BIRCH

My Babcia Halinka could never resist hugging a birch tree, and I take after her. If you place your head against its smooth white trunk, it will bring you a sense of calm and joy, such is the energy of the birch. In the past, the birch energy was equated to that of children.

The ancient Slavs drank birch water, and this is something that is still practised in the Baltic States to this day. I love birch water; it's not only delicious and refreshing but also life-affirming and deeply regenerating. However, to tap the tree you need to know exactly what you are doing in order not to harm or kill it, so I prefer to leave that ritual to the experts.

During the spring festival of *Zielone Świątki* – the Green Holiday – birch branches were used to bring spring into the household, thus ensuring a good harvest, prosperity and abundance. Birch's delicate, young branches were also used to whack the cattle (more of a massage really), ensuring good health for the year. You might still encounter a birch slapping should you find yourself in a traditional Slavic bath house, for they are reputed to improve circulation and energy levels.

BIRCH MASSAGE to improve energy levels and circulation

If you don't have the opportunity to go to a traditional bath house, you can create your own at home, and give yourself a birch (*Betula pendula*) massage for good health. You will get to control the strength with which you apply the branches, rather than being at the mercy of a Slavic bathhouse devotee.

Note:
Cut the branches where there is a natural swelling.

About 13 small birch branches
Natural string

◉ Trim the birch branches to about 20cm (8in) in length. Tie the branches together at the bottom with the string. Wrap with enough string to produce a clear handle.

◉ Take a warm, steamy shower, and gently beat the birch branches against your skin, from your feet, up your legs, toward the heart. Then down your arms, along your collarbone and down your back.

◉ Wash yourself and finish with a cold shower.

VODKA INFUSED WITH YOUNG WALNUTS for any stomach complaint

My Babcia Ziuta always had a bottle of *orzechówka* – walnut vodka medicine – on hand for those suffering from indigestion or simply over-eating, which was very easily done at her house, as she was a cook by profession and a feeder by nature. This vodka is a great remedy and digestif, yet the taste has always been unpleasant to say the least – it's very bitter! It was considered a necessary evil.

My mum has greatly improved this recipe with the addition of honey, cinnamon and cloves, but please remember this is still a medicine and not a liquor. My mother says that walnuts (*Juglans regia*) act like antibiotics in this form. I take half a shot of this when needed.

MAKES AROUND 65 DOSES

DOSAGE: Up to 1 x 30ml/1fl oz shot (2 tablespoons) whenever you feel a stomach complaint coming on.

40–50g/1½–1¾oz green, unripe walnuts (picked in June)
1l/35fl oz/4¼ cups good-quality vodka
1l/35fl oz/4¼ cups good-quality honey
1 cinnamon stick
10–15 cloves
3l/100fl oz sterilized glass jar
2l/70fl oz sterilized glass bottle

◉ Rinse the walnuts under running water. Halve them and place in the jar.

◉ Cover with the vodka. Place the lid loosely on the jar and leave in a warm spot (a sunny windowsill is ideal). Leave to ferment for 2 weeks, stirring every day.

◉ After 2 weeks, strain the walnuts out. Mix the liquid with the honey.

◉ Place the cinnamon stick and cloves in the glass bottle. Pour in the vodka medicine. Seal with the lid and leave for 6 months to a year.

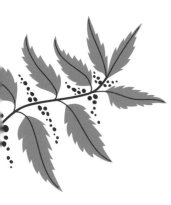

WOODLAND STEW WITH NETTLES AND WILD MUSHROOMS
for all ills

A simple, warming stew is perfect for those chilly days of spring, when the nettles have finally appeared in the woods and everything is essentially emerging from hibernation.

Nettles (*Urtica dioica*) are said to be beneficial for the kidneys and urinary tract, to lower blood pressure and reduce inflammation. Some say that nettles have all the nutrients a human body needs. While other babushkas would make salads and soups as a pleasant way of benefitting from this miraculous plant, my Babcia Halinka would beat her legs with nettles in order to improve her circulation.

Mushrooms have also been proven to contain a host of health benefits (some even contain vitamin D), so together, nettles and mushrooms have everything covered. You can increase the vitamin D in fresh mushrooms by leaving them outside in the sun for 30 minutes to an hour.

When picking nettles, take only the top six to eight fresh-looking leaves and don't pick any plants that have flowered; 200g (7oz) of nettle leaves is basically your average tote bag, half full of nettle tops. If it's June and you have found some nettles that haven't started to flower (in a shady area), then you can still make this stew, but I advise that you eat only the leaves, as the stems are fibrous at this time of the year.

I always pick up the dried (though not too dry) sausages that I use for this from a Polish shop. *Myśliwska, toruńska* or *wiejska* all work really well.

SERVES 4-6

50g/1¾oz dried mushrooms, preferably boletus or porcini
1 onion, chopped
4 tablespoons cold-pressed rapeseed/canola oil
2 carrots, diced
30g/1oz celeriac/celery root, peeled and grated or 1 celery stick, chopped

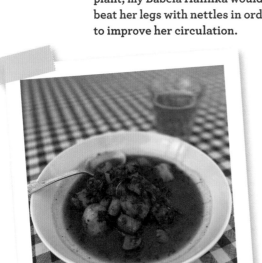

200g/7oz dried sausage, diced
500g/1lb 2oz new potatoes, halved
100g/3½oz chanterelle or chestnut/
    cremini mushrooms, cleaned
    and diced
1 tablespoon butter (salted or
    unsalted)
200g/7oz young nettle tops
100g/3½oz/1¾ cups broad/
    fava beans or frozen peas
3 garlic cloves
2 teaspoons mild mustard (such
    as Polish sarepska mustard)
1 tablespoon chopped fresh dill
Juice of ½ lemon
Salt and black pepper
Crusty bread, to serve

◉ First, rehydrate the dried mushrooms by placing them in a sieve, pouring boiling water over them to open their caps and washing them thoroughly under cold water. Place them in a bowl and pour more boiling water over them. Cover the bowl with a plate and leave for about 30 minutes.

◉ Soften the onion in the oil for a couple of minutes in a saucepan, then add the carrots and celeriac or celery, stir and fry for a further minute. Add the dried sausage, cover the pan and leave to sweat for about 5 minutes. Add the potatoes, stir and cover once more.

◉ Meanwhile, in a separate pan, fry the fresh mushrooms in the butter until golden brown. Set aside.

◉ Place the nettles in a sieve and wash them under running water, then pour some boiling water over them. Transfer to a food processor and blitz a few times. Add these to the main pan with the onion, carrots, sausage, potatoes and celeriac or celery.

◉ Add both the rehydrated mushrooms, with most of their water (leave the last bit, as this might have sediment), and the fried mushrooms to this pan.

◉ Add the broad beans or frozen peas and cover everything with filtered water.

◉ A little trick my grandma used to add flavour to savoury dishes: use the wide edge of a large knife to crush the garlic with some salt. Chop and crush until you get a paste, then add this to the pan. Cover and allow to cook over a low heat for about 30 minutes.

◉ Add the mustard, dill and lemon juice, and season with salt and pepper. Serve with crusty bread.

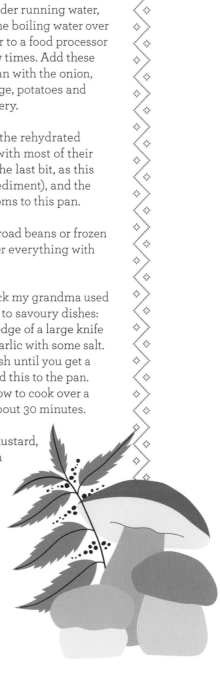

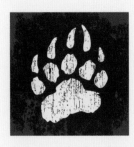

THE BEAR

In the 9th century, Byzantine historians stated that "in a barbaric land of the Slavs, people worship bears as gods, and bears live among humans and roam their settlements". While this may not have been entirely correct, it is certainly true that the bear is a spirit animal to many Slavs.

I once had a dream that I was a huge brown bear. It was so vivid that I've always remembered it. I was down in a hole in the ground, jumping as high as I could, trying to climb out. Finally, gathering all my resources and focusing my strength, I made it out of the bear pit. Apart from drawing my attention to my life situation at the time and what I needed to do to improve it, the dream also highlighted my strong affiliation with bears.

In one Polish folk tale, a bear saves a girl from dying in the forest when she is abandoned there by her weak-willed father at the behest of her wicked stepmother. As usual in folk tales, there are many tests to overcome, but once the girl proves herself to be strong, smart and kind, she is given unlimited riches. In this story, it turns out that the bear was, in fact, a prince turned into an animal.

The bear was considered so powerful in ancient times that his very name was taboo, as was the case with some gods and demons. It was believed by many that bears had the intelligence of humans with super-human strength. In some areas, it was forbidden to eat bear meat, while in other parts, people ate it as part of sacrificial rituals and rites.

The bear is associated with Veles, the ancient God of the Forest (as is the wolf). While Veles was demonized when the Slavic lands turned to Christianity (the horns didn't help), his cult was so omnipotent – all Slavic tribes recognized Veles – that in many places, he was turned into a saint. In Croatia, Veles became Saint Vlaho, the patron Saint of Dubrovnik, while in Russia he became Sanit Vlasiy, who, ironically, took care of sheep and cattle rather than being a wild shapeshifter.

BOSNIAN BEAR PAWS WITH WALNUTS for a healthy mind

To the French, it may be a madeleine, but to a Bosnian, this shape is undoubtedly a bear paw. These crunchy cookies, *šape*, are eaten at every celebratory occasion. The ingredients are simple, yet the recipe varies from one household to the next. They will nevertheless always contain walnuts. Scientists say that eating two walnuts a day can improve brain function (in the olden days, they could have told you that just by looking at the brain-like walnut), so perhaps we should all be eating these golden, melt-in-your-mouth paws to keep our brains in good health. My daughter doesn't like nuts but she loves these, as does everyone else in my family, so a tray like this disappears in one sitting.

MAKES 12 BEAR PAWS

75g/2½oz salted butter, softened
80g/2¾oz/1 cup caster/superfine
    sugar
1 teaspoon vanilla extract
5 tablespoons cold-pressed
    rapeseed/canola oil, sunflower oil
    or olive oil
1 large egg
Zest of 1 lemon
75g/2½oz/½ cup walnuts (crushed)
150g/5½oz/generous 1 cup plain/all-
    purpose flour, plus extra for the tin

1 teaspoon baking powder
Icing/confectioners' sugar, to dust
12-mould madeleine pan

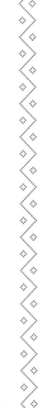

◎ In a food processor or blender, mix the butter, sugar and vanilla together on a high speed until creamy. On a slow speed, gradually add the oil. Add the egg, lemon zest and walnuts.

◎ In a large bowl, whisk the flour and baking powder together.

◎ Slowly pour the butter mixture into the flour mixture, combining until the ingredients are just incorporated. Cover and chill in the refrigerator for 10–15 minutes.

◎ Preheat the oven to 180°C/350°F/Gas mark 4. Grease the madeleine pan and sprinkle with a little bit of flour.

◎ Place a tablespoon of batter in each mould. Bake for 15–17 minutes until golden and slightly crispy.

◎ Cool in the moulds, then remove gently with the help of a spatula. Dust with icing sugar before serving.

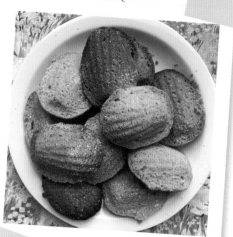

BEAR'S GARLIC TART for much-needed early spring immunity

Mother Nature gives us wild garlic (*Allium ursinum*) – or bear's garlic, as it's called in Poland – at a time in the year when we need it most: the start of spring, when our winter-weary bodies need an immunity boost. Garlic is known for its antibacterial and antiviral properties, and wild garlic is said to have even more of those properties, despite its taste not being as intense. We can eat the leaves and the flowers of wild garlic, so of course we use the flowers to decorate the tart. It's immediately recognizable by its mild garlicky smell, but please always double check if foraging.

I tend to make my own puff pastry, as I find it meditative and calming, but you can of course use ready-made puff pastry if you'd rather – you'll need enough to fill a baking tray.

SERVES 4

FOR THE PUFF PASTRY
250g/9oz/2 cups plain/all-purpose flour, plus extra for dusting
¼ teaspoon salt
150ml/5fl oz/⅔ cup cold water
225g/8oz cold butter (salted or unsalted)

FOR THE TOPPING
200g/7oz/4 cups mixed seasonal mushrooms, roughly chopped
1 tablespoon butter (salted or unsalted)
150g/5½oz wild garlic leaves with stems, plus a few wild garlic flowers, to decorate
150ml/5fl oz/⅔ cup extra virgin olive oil
50g/1¾oz/½ cup grated Parmesan/ pecorino cheese
1 egg, lightly beaten
Sea salt and freshly ground pepper

◙ To make the pastry, put the flour and salt into a food processor and start to blend while you pour in the cold water. As soon as the dough comes together, remove it from the processor, wrap in cling film/plastic wrap and place in the refrigerator for at least 30 minutes.

◙ Place the butter in between two pieces of greaseproof/wax paper and soften it by tapping it with the side of a rolling pin. Cut it in half and place one half on top of the other then reshape it into the size of a large envelope.

◙ Flour your surface and roll the dough into a rough circular shape, about 25cm (10in) in diameter.

◙ Place the butter in the centre of the pastry and fold over the right and left parts of the circle so that they overlap in the middle.

◙ Now, roll the dough into a long rectangle. Mark it into thirds and make a little parcel by folding in the dough from the top to cover the middle third and in the same way from the bottom (over the top).

◙ Do a quarter turn and roll into a long rectangle, then repeat the parcel-making process – into three, down from the top and up from the bottom. A quarter turn and repeat the rolling and parcel-making process once more. Cover in cling film and chill in the refrigerator for about 20 minutes.

◙ Take the dough out of the refrigerator and repeat the parcel-making process a few more times. I enjoy this process, so I repeat it about 10 times, but you could get away with four or five. Chill the dough once again for at least an hour.

◙ In the meantime, fry the mushrooms in the butter until golden. Allow to cool to room temperature before using.

◙ Preheat the oven to 200°C/ 400°F/Gas mark 6.

◙ Remove the flowers of the wild garlic and set aside. Wash the leaves under cold running water, then dry them on a paper towel. Cut the stems off. Discard the ends of the stems, about 5cm (2in), and

chop the rest roughly. Place in a food processor, add 50g (1¾oz) of the leaves and blitz them with the olive oil and a little salt. Add the Parmesan and blitz a few more times to a thin pesto consistency.

◙ Roll out the puff pastry to a rectangle 4mm (¼in) thick and place on a baking sheet. Create a border all the way round by lightly scoring with a knife 2cm (¾in) from the edge. Glaze the edge of the pastry with the egg wash.

◙ Arrange the mushrooms and wild garlic leaves on top of the pastry. Drizzle over the wild garlic pesto and grind over some black pepper.

◙ Bake the tart until the edges of the pastry are golden brown, puffed, and crisp – around 20 minutes.

◙ Let it cool for 5 minutes before cutting it into pieces and serving with some wild garlic flowers on top.

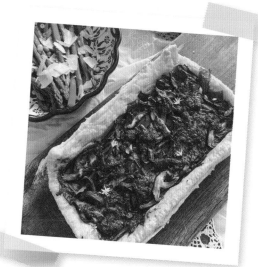

THE IMPORTANCE OF AN EGG

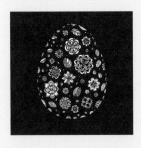

First, there was a golden egg, which hatched in the darkness. Out of that egg came Rod, who, out of loneliness, created the Goddess of Love, Lada. The eggshell cracked and out of it spilled love and light. Since everything was one, Rod had to separate the light from darkness. He created Earth to separate the heavens from the oceans.

This Slavic creation myth (it's not the only one) illustrates the importance of the egg within the Slavic cultures. As the beginning of new life, it is treated as something very special. *Pisanki* – also referred to as *pysanky* or *pisanice* – are the decorated eggs that the Slavs use in Easter rituals. In the olden days, they were strictly the women's domain and if a man walked into the room while they were being decorated, a special cleansing ritual involving salt had to be performed. A clever way of getting some quality time with the girls, perhaps?

Different regions of each country have different types of traditional patterns, decorations and techniques for *pisanki*. Some say that the further East we go, the more intricate the designs. I have always had a soft spot for the *pisanki* from the Kurpie region of Poland, which my grandma Halinka had in her treasure trove of a flat. They had holes in the top and bottom, of course, because "forever *pisanki*" can't have a real egg inside, so the egg is blown out of them. They were light and velvety because they were decorated with wool and the inside of a bulrush plant (as the decorations were stuck and not painted, they were officially *oklejanki*, see page 66), which is a beautiful creamy colour. The end result makes me think of whipped cream on top of a cake. "Forever *pisanki*" are given as gifts in order to bring luck and prosperity to their owner. Historically, one of the most popular ways of decorating them has been batik: using wax to draw patterns, before dying the eggs in darker shades and repeating, until we obtain a multi-layered, cosmic design. Only once the wax has been melted, does the final design reveal itself!

After banning *pisanki* originally, the Church reversed the ban in the 12th century and has now fully embraced this folkloric custom. In Poland, *pisanki* eggs are placed in a basket with other food, such as dried sausage, bread, salt and pepper, as well as spring branches and fluffy chicks or a sugar sheep. The elaborate basket from each household is taken to Church to be blessed, before we begin Easter breakfast and the celebrations can start. The holy eggs are then cracked open and shared amongst the family members with blessings.

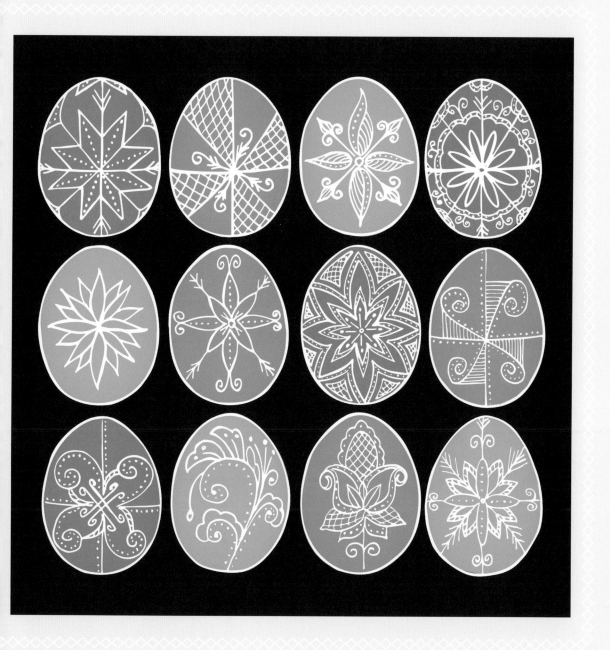

PISANKI IDEAS for Easter

It wouldn't be Easter if we didn't decorate our eggs; it's not something that we are experts in, we just see it as a fun family activity. Therefore, there are all kinds of *pisanki* that we can create with boiled eggs, which are then blessed before we eat them and wish one another good things for the year. If you are interested in serious *pisanki* making, then there are experts who teach some wonderful styles. I suggest you start with these as a fun Easter-time activity to see if you would like to delve deeper into this fascinating art.

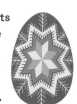

NATURE'S DESIGNS

These are the types of *pisanki* we are accustomed to doing in our family home, as they are fun and not too tricky or time-consuming, and they produce delicate, natural designs. This is very easy to do with small children and choosing interesting leaves is a fun activity in itself. Natural dyes you can use include yellow and red onion skins, red cabbage (if you add bicarbonate of soda the dye will become blue), various tree barks (yellow from an apple tree, for example) and walnut shells to create a dark chocolate brown.

Natural-dye plant matter
Small leaves or flowers
Eggs (as many as you'd like
    to decorate)
An old, very fine sock or nylon
    tights with the feet cut off

◉ Extract the dye from the plant matter by placing it in a saucepan, covering with water and cooking over a medium heat until it comes to the boil. Turn the heat down and simmer for 30 minutes. Each colour needs a separate pan.

◉ Stick a leaf or flower onto the eggs using your saliva and place the sock or tights tightly over the top to hold it in place.

◉ Add the eggs to the pan with the dye using a spoon, so as not to burn yourself.

◉ After about 10 minutes, turn the heat off and leave the eggs in the dye until it cools.

◉ Remove the eggs from the pan and remove the sock or tights. You should have a leaf design on each egg.

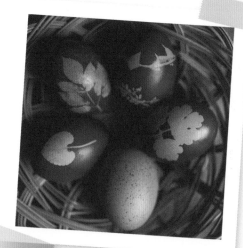

PISANKI DRAPANKI

This was a favourite method in our family house until my children came along. All of a sudden, we realized it's quite hard and time-consuming from a child's perspective, not to mention easy to hurt yourself, as you need to use a sharp object.

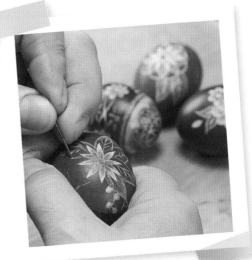

Eggs (as many as you'd like to decorate)
Natural-dye plant matter (see page opposite)
Sharp utensil such as the end of a knife

◉ First, dye the eggs in various dyes – using natural ones is best!

◉ Then use a sharp utensil to scratch patterns onto the eggshell. This takes time and patience, but the results can be rather lovely.

PISANKI OKLEJANKI

This type of *pisanki* is popular in the villages near Kraków, where colourful folk designs are cut out of paper and stuck onto the eggs. Popular designs include the rooster, leaves and flowers. In other areas, wool, materials and even dried plants are used to decorate the eggshells. As we blow the egg out first, the eggshell is very delicate, so this method is aimed at adults and possibly older children (12 plus).

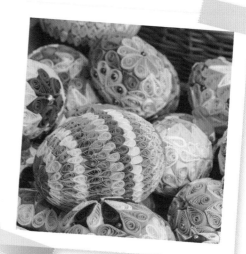

Fine, colourful paper of various colours
Sharp scissors
Strong glue
Un-boiled, white eggs (as many as you'd
    like to decorate)

◉ Draw and cut out bold shapes – big and small. For example, cut out some blue and red flowers, then plenty of smaller coloured circles and small green leaves.

◉ Select your favourite shapes and stick them on the eggs in a pattern of your own creation, layering them to create more elaborate effects.

PISANKI MALOWANKI

Malowanki are painted *pisanki*. If you would like to use boiled eggs, which are later eaten, we need to make sure that the paint we use is completely safe.

The instructions below are for "forever *pisanki*" that are given as gifts rather than eaten. There are many techniques to paint the eggshells – some like to split the *pisanki* into sections and sketch designs on with a pencil first, before painting one section at a time. If you would like to do this, you can make the sketch first, before blowing. Needless to say, you need to hold the empty eggshell very carefully.

Un-boiled eggs (as many as you'd like
   to decorate)
Acrylic paints and paintbrushes or
   acrylic paint pens

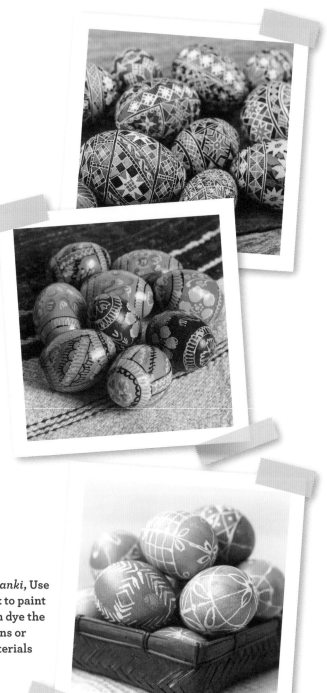

◙ With a needle or pin, make a hole on the top and bottom of each egg. Place your lips to one of the holes and blow all the egg out over a bowl.
◙ First, paint the entire eggshell any colour of your choosing. Allow to dry.
◙ Paint natural designs onto your eggs, allowing each side to dry before starting on the next.

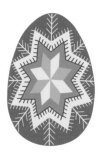

PISANKI BATIQUE

To make simple batique *pisanki*, Use a toothpick and melted wax to paint a design into your egg, then dye the egg natually with onion skins or any of the other dyeing materials mentioned on page 64.

DEVILLED EGGS WITH SALMON ROE, for love and fertility

As a symbol of new life, fertility and prosperity, there cannot be a Slavic Easter celebration without devilled eggs. Each home has their own particular recipe, though, and mine is slightly unusual in that we make an egg paste using lovage (*Levisticum officinale*) for love. I feel that this is in tune with the old Slavic ways. Lovage was the herb most used for love potions in the past, and it will probably come as no surprise that love potions were the most common reason why people would turn to magic for help. In the UK, dried lovage is easily accessible from any Polish shop (name: *lubczyk*).

Note:
When I say something is for fertility, it is, of course, symbolic and not a cure for fertility problems.

SERVES 10–12

12 eggs, hard-boiled and peeled, then halved
5 tablespoons mayonnaise
1 teaspoon mild mustard (such as sarepska or Dijon)
2 teaspoons finely chopped fresh lovage, or 1 teaspoon dried
1 teaspoon finely chopped fresh chives
1 teaspoon finely chopped fresh dill
½ teaspoon salt
¼ teaspoon white pepper
Salmon roe, to decorate

◉ Scoop the yolks out of the eggs into a mixing bowl, then add the mayonnaise and mustard and mix to combine. Add the herbs, salt and white pepper and mix thoroughly.

◉ Scoop the filling back into the eggs and finish them off with ¼ teaspoon of salmon roe on top of each (more eggs for extra fertility and prosperity).

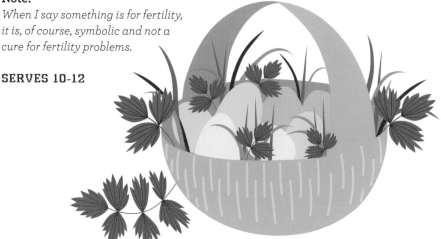

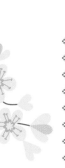

MAY HAWTHORN FLOWER *NALEWKA* to calm the nerves and lower blood pressure

The subtle hawthorn flowers have treasure hidden within their delicate petals, it's just a matter of knowing and preserving ...

In the north of Poland, there is a special name for a *nalewka* – medicinal vodka – made from the flowers of hawthorn (*Crataegus monogyna*): *bulimączka*, which shows its popularity in the area. It is thought to calm the nerves and lower blood pressure, as well as help strengthen the heart. You can also make *nalewka* from hawthorn berries, incidentally, but I prefer this delicate, floral recipe.

We pick the hawthorn flowers before midday and before they are in full bloom. There should be a lot of buds and a few smaller leaves are fine too.

If you would like to use this as a medicine, then drink half a shot (1 tablespoon) a day for a couple of weeks, then take a break for a month before repeating (always consult with your medical practitioner first, to make sure that it won't affect you adversely).

MAKES ABOUT 48 DOSES

50 hawthorn flowers and buds (approximately)
500ml/17fl oz/2 cups good-quality vodka
200ml/7fl oz/scant 1 cup good-quality runny honey
1l/35fl oz sterilized glass jar
1l/35fl oz sterilized glass bottle

◉ Wash the hawthorn flowers and buds very gently and allow to dry on paper towels.

◉ Place the flowers in the sterilized jar and cover with the vodka. Close the lid and place in a cool, dark spot for 2 weeks, either stirring or shaking lightly once a day.

◉ After 2 weeks, strain out the flowers and add the runny honey (if it's not very runny, then warm it gently first).

◉ Transfer to the sterilized bottle, seal with the lid and allow to stand for 3–6 months (or longer) before using.

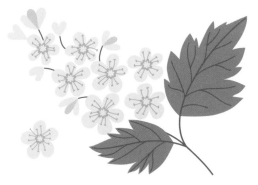

BLACK RADISH SYRUP
for a sore throat

My mum taught me to make this syrup almost as an afterthought. She happened to come across a black radish at the market and remembered what her mother used to do with it. This syrup does wonders to soothe a sore throat – take 1 tablespoon two or three times a day.

MAKES 1 X 100ml/3½fl oz BOTTLE

1 round black radish
100ml/3½fl oz/scant ½ cup good-
   quality runny honey
100ml/3½fl oz sterilized glass bottle

◙ Wash and dry the black radish and, using a sharp knife and spoon, scoop out the middle. You want to make a deep hole, about three-quarters the length of the radish and about 5cm (2in) across if possible. Leave about 5cm (2in) of radish flesh around the edge.

◙ Pour the honey into the hole. Loosely cover to prevent dirt from getting in and leave at room temperature for 1 week, then transfer to the bottle. Screw the lid on and keep in your cupboard for up to 2 months.

RASPBERRY LEAF INFUSION to support fertility or ease perimenopause

A cup of raspberry leaf tea a day is often recommended to pregnant women to strengthen the womb lining. If you are trying for a baby, then you could start earlier, as they also support fertility. Nowadays, I drink raspberry leaf infusion to ease the symptoms of perimenopause. The young, vibrant leaves are best, therefore collect in spring and dry them for the future.

To dry:

1. *Spread the leaves out on a rack and dry in a warm, shaded place for a week. Transfer to a paper bag.*
2. *Spread the leaves out on a tray lined with baking paper and place in the oven at the lowest setting, leaving the door ajar. Turn them every 20 minutes. Depending on how many you have, this should take 2–3 hours. Turn the heat off and allow them to continue drying in the warm oven for another hour. Transfer to a paper bag.*

MAKES 1 INFUSION

7 dried raspberry leaves
1 teaspoon good-quality honey

◙ Place the leaves in a cup and pour over the hot (not boiling) water. Cover with a saucer and allow to infuse for 5–10 minutes.

◙ Sweeten with honey and drink daily.

LADY OF THE WOOD
(A Czech–Slovak story)

Cheerful Betushka and her mother were poor and lived in a tumbledown cottage near a birch wood with their two nanny goats. From spring to autumn, Betushka would go out to the pasture with her goats, and every day her mother handed her a basket with a slice of bread and a spindle in it. "Bring home a full spindle", she always said. While Betushka worked hard for her mother, she loved nothing more than to dance.

One day at noon, just after she had eaten and was getting up to have her usual dance around, a beautiful lady appeared in front of her. She was draped in a white dress as fine as a spider's web and on her head was a wreath of woodland flowers. "Come, let us dance together", she said.

Enchanting music sounded overhead as all the woodland birds came to sit upon the birch branches and sang for them. As Betushka danced, she forgot her spinning and her goats. Only when the sun went down did the music cease. Betushka realized she hadn't completed her work and hid her spindle and flax in the bottom of the basket, hoping to make up for it the next day.

The next day, when noon came, Betushka ate her bread, giving the goats her leftovers, then ran off to collect some berries. When she returned, she decided to have a quick dance before continuing her work. However, as soon as she began, the Lady of the Wood appeared once again. This time Betushka said: "Forgive me, Lady, but I cannot dance today, I must do my work."

The beautiful maiden replied, "Come Betushka, let's dance. Before the sun goes down, I will help you spin your flax."

So, for the second time, the musicians in the treetops started their music and Betushka and the Lady danced together. Betushka could not take her eyes off the enchanting maiden as they whirled. The whole day passed as if in a trance. Then the sun went down and Betushka burst into tears. "My mother will scold me for this."

The Lady took the flax from her head, wound it round the stem of a birch and began to spin. Before the sun sank all the flax was spun.

"Reel, and grumble not!", she said and vanished.

The next day, when the sun was at its highest, Betushka laid her spindle on the grass, gathered some blueberries, then jumped up to dance. Again, the Lady appeared. She smiled at Betushka, put her arm about her, and as the music above their heads began to play, they whirled round and round. When they stopped the sun was already set behind the woods. Betushka burst into tears.

"Give me your basket", the Lady said, "and I will put something in it

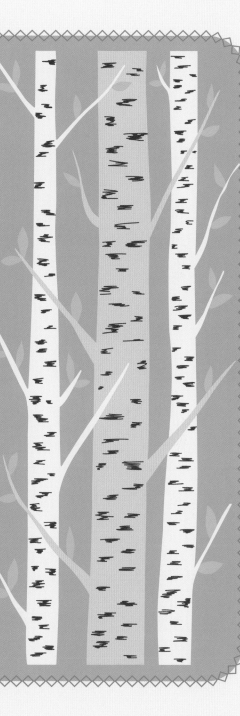

to make up for today, but look not inside until you're home." And she was gone.

The basket was so suspiciously light that Betushka wondered whether there was anything in it at all, so halfway home, she peeped in. It was full of birch leaves! Betushka reproached herself for being so gullible. In her vexation she threw out a handful of leaves, but then thought: "I'll keep what's left for the goats."

She was almost afraid to go home, but her mother was waiting.

"Betushka, what kind of a spool did you bring home yesterday?"

"Why?" Betushka replied nervously.

"This morning, I reeled and reeled and the spool remained full. 'What evil spirit has spun that?' I cried out impatiently, and instantly the yarn disappeared from the spindle as if blown away."

Betushka confessed everything. "That was a Lady of the Wood!" her mother cried. "At noon and midnight the wood maidens dance. It is well you are not a little boy or she might have danced you to death, but they are often kind to little girls. Why didn't you tell me? If I hadn't grumbled, I could have had enough yarn to fill the house!"

Betushka thought of her basket and ran to have another look. The birch leaves had turned into pure, shining gold!

Betushka reproached herself: "She told me not to look inside until I got home, but I didn't obey."

Nevertheless, the riches that Betushka had brought home were enough for her mother to buy a farm with cattle. Betushka had pretty clothes and no longer had to look after goats all day. But no matter what she did, no matter how cheerful she was, nothing ever gave her quite so much pleasure as dancing with the Lady of the Wood.

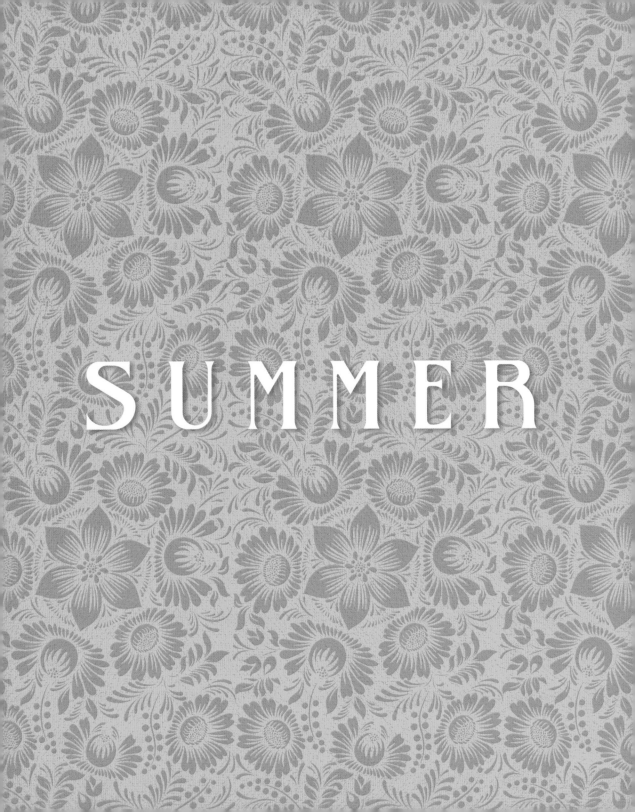

SUMMER

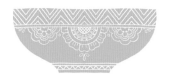

Summer glistens in the lakes, rivers and seas of Eastern Europe. It's the smell of pine and wild flowers and of skin that's been warmed by the sun. It's sitting under fruit trees in someone's garden with the sound of crickets all around, then noisy dogs barking late into the night (certainly more Slavic in temperament). It's the taste of soft fruit, picked and eaten there and then. It's also the taste of cool fruit soup, pasta with berries and yeasty buns with fruit in the middle.

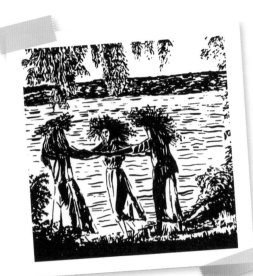

The Slavic celebration of Midsummer is called Kupala Night – an ancient festival that still takes place in Poland, Ukraine, Belarus and beyond ... In the past, this was a feral night of free love and fire jumping, fortune telling and wild swimming. There is a myth that a magical fern flower appears at midnight and will grant you any wish should you find it. While the night will always be joyous and ethereal, it's certainly a less raucous affair now than that of old. Nevertheless, the link to fertility and purification stands, because fire and water are both means of purifying, and we all feel that connection deep within our psyche. Even if you are not celebrating in a group, you could have a private celebration by going for a wild swim, making a wildflower wreath or cooking your food on an open fire outdoors. You could even go on a midnight woodland walk to search for that elusive fern flower.

If there has been enough rain during spring, the crops will be doing well and the people will be satisfied. However, if spring has been dry, the people will be worried and it will be time for the rites of Dodola. Dodola was one of the most significant deities in Slavic mythology and the wife of the Thunder God, Perun. Of this union, Dziewanna, the Hunter Goddess, was born. Alas, Slavic deities didn't tend to be monogamous and when Dodola was seduced by Veles (Volos), the God of the Wild Animals, Water and the Underworld, she gave birth to the God of the Spring Sun, Yarilo. Dodola was known by many names: Perperuna, Dzidzila, Vyasna-Vyasnyanka (alluding to spring in Belarussian), Letnica (alluding to summer in Polish) and Molonya (alluding to thunder in Ukrainian). Since the Southern Slavs had a warmer climate, the rites of Dodola took on a special urgency and needed to be performed often. In Serbian villages, one teenage girl was wrapped in garlands of green and, accompanied by a group of children, she went from one house to another, spinning and dancing. On each doorstep the lady of the house would pour water on her while they all chanted:

Fall, O rain! and gentlest dew!
    Oy, Dodo! Oy, *Dodole!*
Refresh our pasture – lands and fields!
    Oy, Dodo! Oy, *Dodole!*

The girl who is chosen to lead the procession would often be an orphan, who would then receive coins and gifts for her service to the community. Gifts of food (nothing round, however, as that could induce hail, according to superstition) would also be bestowed upon the procession and all the children would feast together afterwards.

The month of August, *sierpień*, is actually named after the sickle in Polish, which makes it clear what this time has historically always been about in the Slavic communities. This is harvest time. A busy, bountiful time of reaping what we have sowed earlier in the year, followed by a celebration. In Polish, it's called *żniwa* and the celebration after the harvest that marks the end of summer is *wyżynki* or *dożynki*, but it has been known by many names in the past. It is a festival of gratitude (to God since Christianity took over) and of bonding. Now the harvest is mainly mechanical, we have somewhat lost that feeling of community during this time. However, there are places that still celebrate in quite elaborate ways by creating all kinds of objects out of straw to display during a procession.

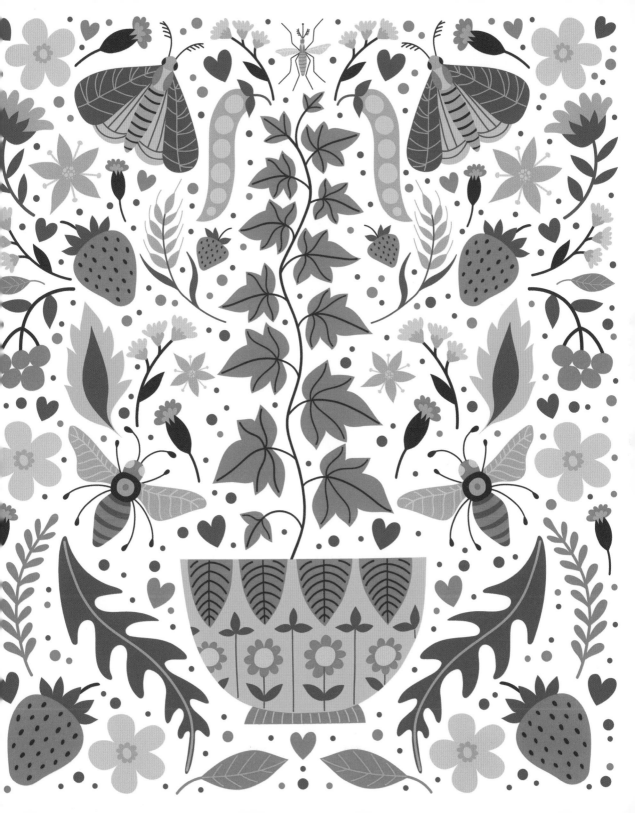

ENERGIZING PEPPERMINT OIL
for a sprightly body and quick mind

This is the perfect way to cool down after a day in the sun, while giving your skin some love and attention. After a cool shower, I massage this oil into my skin while it's still wet. Then I pat my skin dry, leaving it hydrated and revived.

Peppermint (*Mentha piperita*) is known to revitalize and cool. There are many types of mint, and while all are suitable, peppermint has the strongest effect and the most cooling sensation.

Cold-pressed sunflower oil contains vitamin E and is known to brighten the skin, so it's a good choice as a carrier oil.

MAKES 1 x 250ml/9fl oz BOTTLE

50 fresh peppermint leaves
150ml/5fl oz/⅔ cup cold-pressed sunflower oil
250ml/9fl oz sterilized glass jar
250ml/9fl oz sterilized glass bottle

SUNSHINE METHOD

◉ Place half of the peppermint leaves in the jar and pour over the oil, making sure all the leaves are covered with oil. Close the lid.

◉ Leave in a warm, sunny spot in your house (a sunny windowsill is perfect) for 7 days to infuse, turning the jar about thrice a day.

◉ After 7 days, strain out the peppermint leaves, pressing all the oil out of them and add a new batch of leaves to the jar. Place these into your sunny spot for another 7 days.

◉ Strain the leaves out and pour the oil into a sterilized glass bottle. Keep in a cool, shady place and use within 2 months.

SPEEDY METHOD

◉ Place half of the peppermint leaves in the jar and pour over the oil, making sure all the leaves are covered with oil. Close the lid.

◉ Place the jar in a medium-sized saucepan over a low heat with around 4cm (1½in) of water. Heat gently for 1.5 hours. Cool slightly before straining the leaves out through a muslin or gauze, pressing all the oil out of them.

◉ Add the next batch of leaves to the jar and heat in the same way.

◉ Strain the leaves out and pour the oil into a sterilized glass bottle. Keep in a cool, shady place and use within 2 months.

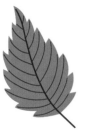

SOOTHING SORREL FACE MASK for a summer's evening

Wonderful as it all is, the summer sun, the salty sea and the grainy sand can leave the more sensitive skins among us with a few minor irritations. This is a mask to soothe those irritations at the end of the day, but also to slow the aging process too (probably due to all that vitamin C and A).

What I love about this mask is that you only need a few sorrel leaves. If you are making the classic Slavic sorrel soup, you need a large bagful or even two, which takes a while to forage and even longer to sort through to make sure you have only lovely sorrel leaves. This is not that kind of all-day affair. I make this mask whenever I see some sorrel growing in the summer (though never by a roadside), whether my skin is feeling irritated or not. I don't always make the full amount; sometimes I just grab a handful as I'm walking past and use a pestle and mortar to break them up if I don't have enough for a food processor. This mask is best applied at night, after a long day in the sun.

Make sure you don't confuse sorrel (*Rumex acetosa*) for cuckoo-pint (*Arum maculatum*), which is toxic and an irritant.

MAKES 5 MASKS

25 young (small) sorrel leaves
10 tablespoons full-fat yogurt

◉ Wash the sorrel leaves, then roughly chop and place in a food processor with the yogurt. Blitz a few times until the sorrel juices are released and the yogurt turns a little green.

◉ Massage about 2 tablespoons of the mask into your face for 1–2 minutes. Leave the mask on for 5–10 minutes, then wash off with cold water. Towel-dry your face and follow with your favourite night oil or cream.

◉ Use this mask every day for 5 days to relieve and soothe your summer skin.

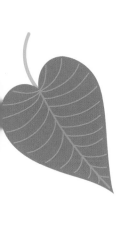

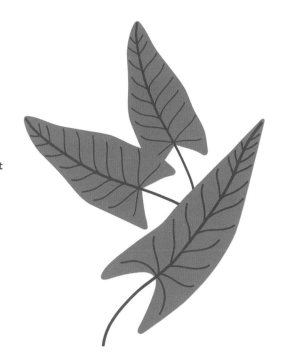

STRAWBERRY FACE MASK for smooth, summer skin

Early summer strawberries speak of sunny days and balmy evenings ahead. Even the bright, heart-shaped appearance of this fruit feels jubilant. Conversely, at any other time of the year, strawberries that are artificially grown and injected into the supermarkets lose their appeal for me. Eating strawberries when they're ripe is the greatest pleasure. Plus, the few overripe, squashed ones needn't feel like a loss, because they are perfect for a face mask that will calm and rejuvenate your skin.

MAKES 1 MASK

2 very ripe, organic
   strawberries
1 tablespoon full-fat yogurt

◎ Place the strawberries in a small bowl and squash them with a fork until they turn to mush.

◎ Add the yogurt to the bowl and continue to mash, until the yogurt turns pink.

◎ Apply this mask to your face and relax for 5–10 minutes before washing off with cold water.

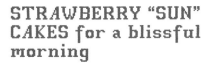

STRAWBERRY "SUN" CAKES for a blissful morning

Just looking at a plump red strawberry takes me to a magical realm, like the one portrayed in the Russian Khokhloma paintings, with vibrant reds and golds popping out against a black background. This painting style was used by the Old Believers, who, fleeing persecution in the 17th century, took refuge in the woods. When their style of painting merged with the art of the local craftsmen who carved wooden objects, the village of Khokhloma started producing striking black, red and gold tableware that is now known all over the world. The mythical glowing Firebird is often depicted in these folk crafts (see page 84).

Strawberries are known to have many health benefits, from supporting heart health to reducing blood sugar and boosting your immunity, but as their skin is very thin, it's important to always choose organic strawberries.

The round shape of drop scones has made them a perfect celebratory Slavic food throughout the ages because the shape was always seen to symbolize the sun. These joyous strawberry "sun" cakes are an ideal way to celebrate the simple things, like a gentle summer's morning. These are perfect for breakfast, brunch or a mid-afternoon snack.

SERVES 4

300g/10½oz/2¼ cups plain/
   all-purpose flour
1½ tablespoons golden caster/
   granulated sugar
Large pinch of salt
1 teaspoon baking powder
2 eggs, separated, plus 2 whites
250ml/9fl oz/1 cup milk (or milk
   alternative)
1 tablespoon cold-pressed
   rapeseed/canola oil (or another
   mild oil), plus extra for frying
½ teaspoon vanilla extract
1 tablespoon sour cream or
   thick kefir
350g/12oz/2 cups strawberries, sliced
Icing/confectioners' sugar
   or honey, to serve

◉ Combine the flour, sugar, salt
and baking powder in a large bowl
and whisk gently to combine (you
can also use a food processor or
blender on a low setting for this).
Add the egg yolks and pour in
the milk while mixing with a
wooden spoon.

◉ Once the batter is smooth,
add the oil, vanilla extract and
sour cream and stir again.

◉ In a separate bowl, beat the
egg whites until they form stiff
peaks. Fold them gently into the
batter. Add the strawberry slices,
reserving some to put on top as
they are frying (about 24).

◉ Heat a thin layer of oil in a
large frying pan and, once hot,
spoon tablespoons of batter into it
(place a drop in first to check – if
it bubbles immediately, then it's
ready). Fry the cakes in batches of
3–4, depending on the size of your
pan – you will need room to turn
them over. Pop a strawberry slice
on the top of each. After about 2–3
minutes (less once your pan gets
really hot), flip them and fry the
other sides for another 2 minutes.
Remove from the pan and set
aside on a paper towel to soak
up any excess oil. In between
batches, give the pan a quick
wipe, then add a bit more oil.

◉ Serve warm, dusted with icing
sugar or drizzled with honey.

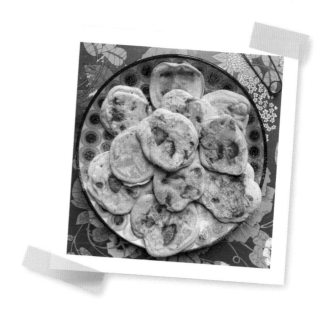

FIREBIRD

With golden feathers that glow like flames as it flies, the mythical Firebird is a longed-for character in many a Slavic folk tale. Often the object of a magical quest, the Firebird can bring both fortune and misfortune, depending on the hero's decisions and intentions.

In the Czech story "The Firebird and the Red Fox", a young prince goes in search of the Firebird in order to bring his ill father good health. He visits many kingdoms and in each one he is given yet another unattainable task. He is helped by a fox, who knows all the secrets of the land. However, the prince has some trouble listening to the fox's instructions and gets himself into all kinds of trouble. Yet the fox, despite being angry, never abandons the prince. He senses his soft heart and has faith. In the end, the prince heals his father, shares his kingdom and marries the princess from the Black Sea that he met along the way.

In the Russian tale "The Firebird and Princess Vasilisa", an archer picks up the Firebird's luminous feather, against his horse's advice, and is set on a series of impossible quests by the capricious king. This time, it is the horse that helps his master with each unattainable task and even protects him from a boiling cauldron with a magical spell. In the end, it is the unreasonable king who is boiled, and the archer takes his place as ruler of the land and marries the magical Princess Vasilisa from the sea.

In each of the tales, the Firebird marks the beginning of a difficult quest. Other similarities include the constant unworkable tasks, the princesses from the sea (linking the feminine to the water element) and the magical animals who help the hero. In both, the hero finds strength he didn't know he had and eventually wins both the crown and love.

The messages of the Firebird stories have felt particularly apt for my writing this book. In my case, the Firebird symbolizes the book itself – something otherworldly and magical that has filled me with awe every time I get into the flow of writing it. Yet, with two young children to look after (the younger one with no childcare), a PhD to work on and a busy working partner, I have found that at times my quest has also felt impossible, and the challenges of everyday life insurmountable. So, what lessons have I learned from the Firebird stories? Resilience – to accept my quest and keep re-accepting it every day. To ask my intuition (the animal) to guide me when I don't know how to proceed. To remain soft and kind, and to allow the magic to flow.

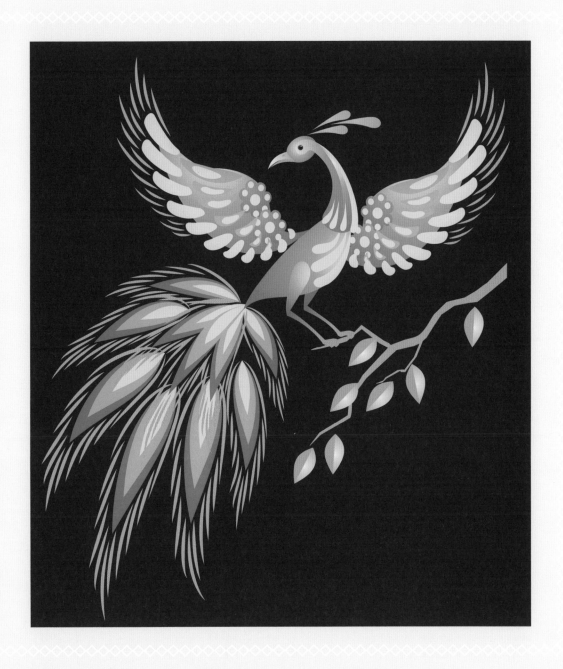

GOLDEN INFUSION for urinary tract health

Tiny sunny flowers beam at us from every field, every garden, every roadside. The wispy yellow Canadian goldenrod (*Solidago canadensis*) has taken over central Poland, and while it's often blamed for allergies, some experts claim its pollen particles are, in fact, too big to cause that reaction and other, less visible plants are to blame instead.

Its name is *nawłoć* in Polish, yet in folklore this plant was known as *złotnik* – "the goldsmith" – among other things. The latin name – *Solidago* – alludes to its healing powers. I have heard of honey made from this common wildflower, yet until recently I have never used it myself. My aunt assured me that the goldenrods have many uses and benefits – it's said to aid digestion, reduce inflammation and act as an antibacterial agent.

All the goldenrods are beneficial to the urinary tract, which I have had issues with in the past, so I drink this golden tea in the summer as part of my prevention method. I have also found that using the infusion (without honey) as a toner makes my skin feel more radiant, so I always brew more for that purpose (it lasts 3 days if you cover it).

Note:
Goldenrod is picked when it's in full bloom and the weather is sunny (and, as always, we need to make sure we know exactly what we are picking).

To dry:
Dry it spaced out on trays in a warm, well-ventilated, shady spot, then store in an airtight container for up to 6 months.

SERVES 2

2 tablespoons fresh goldenrod flowers, or 1 tablespoon dried
400ml/14fl oz/1²/₃ cups hot water from a pre-boiled kettle
2 teaspoons good-quality honey

◉ Wash the flowers under running water, then place into a large mug or a small teapot. Pour the hot water over the flowers, cover the mug or teapot and allow to infuse for 5–10 minutes.

◉ Add honey to sweeten and mix well. Strain the flowers out before drinking (my teapot strains them for me).

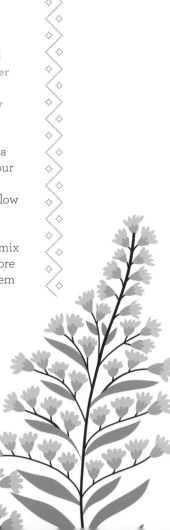

FERMENTED PEAS AND RADISHES to lower cholesterol

Fermenting has been used throughout the ages in Slavic countries to preserve food. It has always been clear to Slavs that fermented foods are beneficial to health because of how they make us feel. The brine often doubled up as a hangover cure too. Modern science has now proven that the fermenting process increases the availability of the nutrients in the food and produces cultures that improve gut health. To me, fermenting is kitchen alchemy at its most powerful. Both these ferments are reputed to lower cholesterol.

MAKES 1 x 250ml /9fl oz JAR

200ml/7fl oz/scant 1 cup warm water from pre-boiled kettle
½ tablespoon sea salt
150g/5½oz radishes, halved, or fresh peas
2 garlic cloves, halved lengthways
2–3 pimento berries
2 leaves from a blackberry, blueberry or raspberry bush
250ml/9fl oz sterilized glass jar

◉ Pour the warm water over the salt and mix until the salt dissolves. Allow to cool for 20-30 minutes until only a little warm.

◉ Place the radishes or peas in your jar along with the garlic, berries and one of the leaves. Pour the slightly warm, salty water over the top and cover with the final leaf. If anything is popping out you could place a small clean pebble wrapped in cling film/plastic wrap on top, or I tend to use a small silicone weight.

◉ Place the jar on a saucer, cover with a dish towel and leave at room temperature for 2-3 days. You can now try the contents and see if you like the taste. If you would like them more fermented, you can leave the jar for another 24 hours. After this, close the lid and keep in the refrigerator.

Note:
If you see any green or black mould (which has happened to me only twice in my entire fermenting life), then throw the contents of the jar out. If you see a bit of white mould, you can scoop that out and discard it. If the fermented veg still smells good then you can use it, but remember to refrigerate afterwards. If there's a lot of white mould, then I would start again.

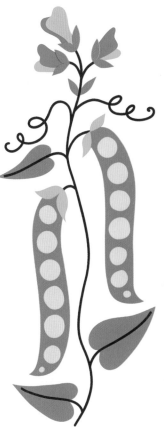

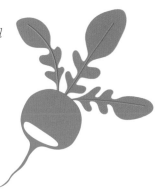

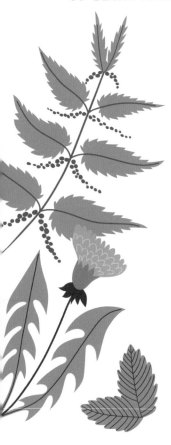

WILD SUMMER PIEROGI for a joyful afternoon of dumpling making and good health

I couldn't resist bringing my two favourite things together in this book – pierogi and wild, foraged foods. As there are so many wild greens in these pierogi (and so many options to mix them up too), it would be difficult to pinpoint exactly what they are good for, as they are basically good for everything! Look for the wild greens growing around your house, because according to some folk practitioners, this is what will be best for you.

Hawthorn (*Crataegus species*) was used by the ancient Slavs to repel demons and diseases (often the same thing in their eyes) and has now been scientifically proven to be beneficial for the heart and cardiovascular system. In folk medicine it has many more uses than that; the old Slavs used hawthorn to help with insomnia, soothe a sore

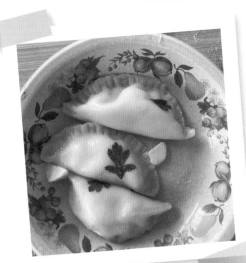

stomach and even relieve asthma. Then there's all the other wild greens ... I like to use a mixture of sorrel (*Rumex acetosa*), wild spinach (*Chenopodium album*) and dandelion (*Taraxacum officinale*) leaves, as well as young nettles in these pierogi – all powerful healing forces. Historically, ground ivy (*Glechoma hederacea*) had been widely used in the Polish kitchen. As a folk medicine, it was used to treat both lung issues and digestive problems, similar to mint, which can be used instead.

As you've probably guessed, you can be flexible on the wild greens you use here – if you can't get the wild sorrel/nettles etc, just use baby spinach; if you can't get hold of either mint or dill, leave them out. You could replace hawthorn with flat leaf parsley too.

SERVES 4

FOR THE DOUGH
300g/10½oz/2¼ cups plain/
    all-purpose flour, plus extra
    for rolling
Large pinch of salt
2 tablespoons cold-pressed
    rapeseed/canola oil
120ml/4fl oz/½ cup warm water
    from a pre-boiled kettle

FOR THE FILLING
30 young hawthorn leaves
20–30 sorrel, wild spinach,
    dandelion or young nettle leaves

150g/5½oz/¾ cup twaróg
   cheese or ricotta
1 egg yolk
10 ground ivy or mint leaves,
   finely chopped
1 teaspoon finely chopped fresh
   dill or fennel fronds
½ teaspoon salt

TO COOK AND SERVE
20g/¾oz salted butter, melted
Sour cream
1 teaspoon salt

◉ Make the dough by combining
the flour and salt in a bowl and
stirring together, then rubbing
the oil in with your fingertips.
Gradually add the water and bring
the dough together with your
other hand. Once the dough has
come together, knead it for 5–6
minutes, then cover with a dish
towel and allow to rest for 20
minutes at room temperature.

◉ Meanwhile, make the filling.
Wash eight of the hawthorn leaves
and finely chop, leaving the rest
whole. Place the sorrel (or spinach/
dandelion/nettle leaves) in a
colander and pour hot (not boiling)
water from a pre-boiled kettle over
them to wilt them. Once they have
cooled, squeeze them with your
hands to release any excess water
before also finely chopping.

◉ Place the twaróg (or ricotta) in
a bowl, then add the egg yolk and
mash together with a fork. Add the
chopped hawthorn, the chopped
sorrel leaves, the ground ivy or
mint, the herbs and the salt to the
bowl and mix well. Set aside.

◉ Bring a large saucepan of water
to the boil. Add 1 teaspoon of salt.

◉ Roll the dough out on a floured
surface, quite thickly at first. Place
the whole hawthorn leaves on the
dough, spacing them out evenly.
Roll the dough thinly now.

◉ Cut circles out of the dough
about 6–7cm (2½in) in diameter,
so that each one has a hawthorn
leaf on it.

◉ Fill each pieróg with a heaped
teaspoon of filling and seal to
make a half moon shape. You can
also use a fork to seal the edges
even more thoroughly. Make sure
they do not touch one another.

◉ Pour the melted butter into
a serving bowl.

◉ Once the water is boiling, cook
the pierogi in batches of five or
six. When they float to the top,
give them another minute before
fishing them out with a slotted
spoon, shaking them gently and
adding straight to the butter bath.

◉ Serve hot with dollops of sour
cream. If you have any left over,
you can fry them the next day
until golden and slightly crispy.

ROSE WATER for a radiant complexion and calm mind

Roses (*Rosa rubiginosa*) have been loved and revered since ancient times for their ornate appearance, soft petals and sweet scent. In Slavic tribes, a rose symbolizes youth, beauty and love.

Different roses smell and taste different, so go by the smell that you like best – and make sure they haven't been sprayed with chemicals. The darker the petals, the more vibrant the colour of the rose water.

This is a general recipe that you can use for both cleansing the face (I like it as a spray) and in cooking. However, I would use distilled water for the face and keep in the refrigerator for up to a month, whereas for cooking, I would use normal water and use it within a week.

MAKES 1 x 350ml/12fl oz JAR

300ml/10½fl oz/1¼ cups water
2 rose heads, red or pink
350ml/12fl oz sterilized glass jar
  or spray bottle

◎ Bring the water to the boil in a small pan, then turn the heat off. Add the rose petals and stir so they are all covered.

◎ Cover the pan and allow the contents to cool to room temperature.

◎ Strain the rose water into your glass jar or bottle and seal it with the lid. Store in the refrigerator.

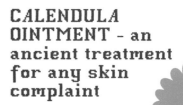

CALENDULA OINTMENT – an ancient treatment for any skin complaint

In my childhood, grey communist blocks would be highlighted with bright-orange pops of the marigolds growing in window boxes. Outside the cities, calendula (more commonly known as "pot marigolds") would be growing in every village garden.

Calendula (*Calendula officinalis*) has been used by Slavs for hundreds of years for its skin-healing properties. It originated in the Mediterranean, and was likely exchanged via the Amber Trail, an ancient trade route which ran from the Baltic countries down the Vistula river in Poland, then south to Rome.

Calendula is known to help any skin complaint, from varicose veins to burns to acne. I've never tested it for acne myself, as I've never had acne and I'm not sure if animal fat would be a good idea to use on it or not. However, I can tell you that in Poland, our ancestors used calendula for everything skin-related and some people still continue to use it today for the same reasons.

MAKES 1 x 120ml/4fl oz JAR

Large handful of calendula/
marigolds (orange) including
petals, leaves, stems, etc.
100g/3½oz/scant ½ cup goose fat
120ml/4fl oz sterilized ointment jar

◉ Gently rinse the calendula
under cold water and allow to
dry naturally. Tear everything
into small pieces.

◉ Heat the goose fat in a frying
pan, then add the calendula
pieces. Cook until they sizzle,
stirring often.

◉ Turn the heat off and allow to
stand for 24 hours, covered, before
heating gently and straining out
the plant matter.

◉ Pour into the jar and keep in
the refrigerator. Use three times a
day when in need.

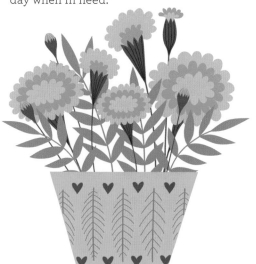

CALENDULA NIGHT BALM for a summer glow

For those of us who feel a bit
squeamish about smearing ourselves
in goose fat, I have devised a night
balm with all the properties of
calendula but no animal fat.

MAKES 2 x 120ml/4fl oz JARS

12–16 fresh calendula/marigolds (orange)
150ml/5fl oz/⅔ cup flaxseed oil
10g/¼oz beeswax
250ml/9fl oz sterilized glass jar
2 x 120ml/4fl oz sterilized jars

◉ Gently rinse the calendula under
cold water and gently pat dry.

◉ Tear into small pieces and place
in the jar. Cover with flaxseed oil.

◉ Place the jar in a saucepan with
around 5cm (2in) of water and simmer.
Leave on a low heat for 2 hours, adding
more water if necessary. Remove from
the heat and cool overnight.

◉ Strain the plant matter out of the oil.

◉ Place the beeswax in a jar and melt
in a saucepan of water over a low heat,
making sure the water covers half the
jar. Once melted, add the marigold oil.
Stir to combine, take off the heat and
cool before pouring into your jars.

◉ Keep at room temperature for
3 months. Use nightly.

THE SACRED LINDEN TREE

If the oak was the sacred male tree to the Slavs, then the linden was the sacred female tree. In Polish, July is called *lipiec*, after the linden tree – *lipa* – which illustrates this tree's importance. Therefore, if you ever see offerings tied to the branches of a linden tree, even if the gifts are Christian in nature (a cross or pictures of saints, for example) this is nevertheless a homage to the old ways. Some linden trees were considered especially important and were thereby mentioned by early historians of the lands. An anonymous monk in the 17th century wrote:

Jest tam w pustynnej miejscowości drzewo nazwane lipą (chiamato Lippa), u którego każdej pierwszej niedzieli dziewiątego księżyca zbiera się mnóstwo Turków i chrześcijan z ofiarami, świecami i innemi rzeczami [...].Oni czczą to drzewo, całują je jak święte relikwje i opowiadają, że tworzy cuda i leczy tych, kto składa mu ofiary [...].

In a deserted village, there is a tree called *lipa* (*Chiamato lippa*), where on the first Sunday of the ninth moon, many Turks and Christians visit with their offerings, candles and the like ... they venerate the tree, kiss it as if it's holy and say it performs miracles and heals those who make it an offering ... (Moszyński, 1934, trans. Zuza Zak)

Loving the linden tree so much, the old Slavs planted them near churches and houses, and near roads so that travellers could rest in their shade. Just touching the trunk of the linden tree was known to be healing. An infusion from its buds and flowers (see page 49) was used to calm the senses and heal colds and sore throats, whereas bathing with linden leaves was said to beautify the body. Additionally, linden was used in ancient beauty products for the face and hair (see opposite for a simple toner).

As linden was considered so healthy, cribs for babies were often made from it, as were many other household utensils and even crosses on graves. Therefore, the linden tree symbolized both fertility and life, as well as both an otherworldliness and a holiness often associated with death.

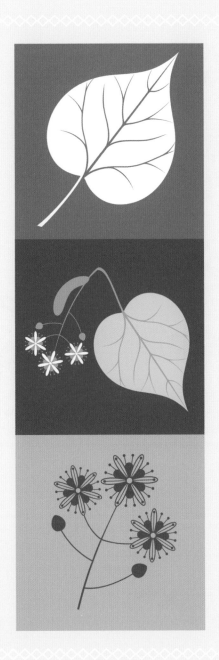

LINDEN FLOWER TONER for soft skin and sacred femininity

The linden tree (genus *Tilia*) is equated with all that is considered to be female – such as beauty and softness – so it's understandable that some Slavs used linden to beautify themselves.

Pick the linden flowers when in bloom, usually around the start of July, and you can dry them for the months to come.

To dry:

Lay the flowers on baking sheets lined with greaseproof/wax paper and place in a warm, well-ventilated but shaded area for 3–4 days. Once dry, transfer to a box with a lid. They should keep for at least 2 months.

MAKES 1 SMALL BOWL

1 tablespoon dried linden flowers
    (or 2 tablespoons if fresh)
150ml/5fl oz/⅔ cup warm
    (not hot) water from a
    pre-boiled kettle

◉ Place the flowers in a bowl and pour the water over them. Cover the bowl with a plate and allow to infuse for at least 20 minutes.

◉ Use this toner with a cotton wool pad, morning and night, for 3 days. Keep covered.

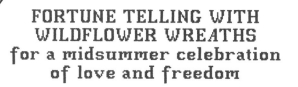

FORTUNE TELLING WITH WILDFLOWER WREATHS
for a midsummer celebration of love and freedom

A field bursting with wild flowers at the height of summer is one of life's joyful sights. The mingling fragrances, the movement of the butterflies and dragonflies, the hum of crickets and bees, all create a hazy, colourful vibration that cannot be captured on a photograph. We can, nevertheless, capture a small portion of this joy in a wild-flower wreath. A wreath is a celebration of youth and the joy, freedom and love it brings.

Wild-flower wreaths used to be made by girls from sacred herbs that grew in the countryside. St John's Wort, the herb that was meant to protect against any malicious natural spirits, was actually known as *Ziele Świętojańskie*, the herb of Midsummer. While opposite you have a list of flowers that are considered to be magical, I would encourage you to choose the ones you are most drawn to when engaging in the making of a wreath.

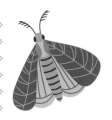

Wild flowers and herbs that are considered to have special powers when used in Slavic wreaths include:

Chamomile
Cornflowers
Mugwort
St John's Wort
Goldenrod
Poppies

Once you have made your wreath and enjoyed wearing it during the day, you need to find some flowing water – a river or stream – for the divination at sunset.

MAKES 1 WREATH

A selection of your favourite wild flowers with long stems

◉ Place two flower heads together and cross the stems. Use one of the stems to wrap around one flower, then around the other flower in a figure of eight movement.

◉ Keep adding flowers and continue using a figure of eight to secure each flower.

◉ To finish, use long grass or a ribbon to secure the two ends and make a circle.

At sunset, head to your nearest river or stream. Get close to the water at a spot where you feel your wreath will have the best chances of a smooth ride. The wreath's journey along the water will reflect the journey of your own love life. If you are doing this in a group, then you should release the wreaths at the same time. The one that is first (it's judged on the journey) will belong to the person who will get married first. If your wreath gets tangled up in reeds, you will not have an easy ride I'm afraid. If you are the slowest, then you will probably marry later in life. Anything else that happens to your wreath may be interpreted as happening to your future romantic life. Take it with a pinch of salt.

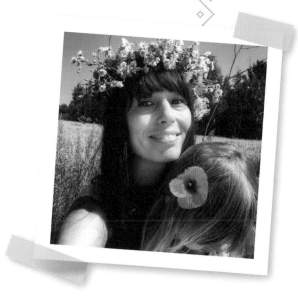

BURDOCK AND NETTLE RINSE for strong, shiny hair

Burdock root (*Arctium*) has been used for strong, shiny hair for hundreds of years, yet ironically I nearly lost my hair trying to pick it. Burdock doesn't come out of the ground easily; if it does, then it could be because the roots are unhealthy, in which case, we don't want that one anyway. However, burdock has prickly burrs, and if, like me, you attempt to pull one that's close to the same height as you, then you are putting yourself at risk of getting them stuck in your hair. I was left with about 26 burrs weaved into an intricate hairstyle, which took over an hour to remove and meant losing clumps of my hair. I don't recommend this route. Go for a healthy green plant that is no taller than your waist and dig around it before pulling the roots out. In the Slavic tradition, burdock root and leaves were collected in July, though in some herbal medicine traditions they are collected after the first frost. Wear gardening gloves and be careful not to bend too close to the plant. You can also buy burdock root very easily online if you would like to avoid the whole process.

If you have managed to collect the burdock yourself, then clean the roots under warm water with a brush (an old toothbrush works well here). Chop them up and dry them out by placing them in the oven at a low temperature (50°C/120°F) for about 3–4 hours. When you want to use them, rehydrate them in some hot water for 2–3 hours.

The stinging nettle (*Urtica dioica*) has been used for hundreds of years for treating hair complaints, so its the perfect companion to burdock for creating strong, healthy hair.

MAKES 1 RINSE

1 tablespoon dried chopped burdock root
20 nettle leaves

◉ Place the burdock root in a saucepan and cover with around 10cm (4in) of water. Bring to the boil, then turn the heat down and simmer for 15 minutes. Turn the heat off.

◉ Add the nettle leaves to the pan, cover and allow to cool.

◉ Strain the nettles and burdock root out of the water.

◉ Use the infused water to rinse your hair after your usual washing routine, as a final step.

◉ This keeps in the refrigerator for up to a week, so you can use it a few times.

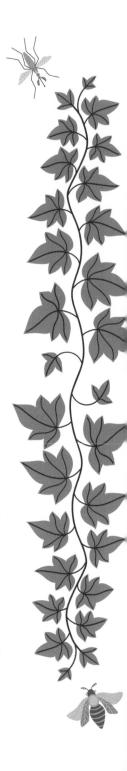

GROUND IVY OIL
for repelling insects the natural way

My aunt Wiesia has pots of ground ivy (*Glechoma hederacea*) hanging down her *dworek* – small manor house – in the Polish town of Ciechocinek. We were staying in a nearby holiday hut once when my aunt's *dworek* had been flooded, and we found many a mosquito lurking about. At night, we heard a buzzing around my daughters' heads and my mum came up with the idea of muddling the ground ivy I had taken from my aunt's and rubbing it on the girls' skin, as well as winding the stems around their bed. None of us got bitten, so I would wholeheartedly recommend ground ivy as a natural insect repellent. I have added lemon peel for its fresh smell and insect repelling properties.

MAKES 1 x 250ml/9fl oz BOTTLE

20 large ground ivy leaves
1 teaspoon grated lemon zest
150ml/5fl oz/⅔ cup cold-pressed flaxseed oil
250ml/9fl oz sterilized glass jar
250ml/9fl oz sterilized glass bottle

NATURAL METHOD

◎ Place all the ingredients in the jar, making sure that the oil covers the leaves and zest. Close the lid and place it on a warm, sunny windowsill. Leave to infuse for 10–14 days.

◎ Strain the leaves and zest out of the oil and pour the oil into a sterilized bottle. Use within 2 months.

SPEEDY METHOD

◎ Place all the ingredients in the sterilized jar, making sure that the oil entirely covers the leaves and zest. Close the lid on the jar and place it in a medium-sized saucepan. Pour around 4cm (1½in) of water into the pan and place over a low heat. Simmer for 1½–2 hours, then turn the heat off and allow to cool.

◎ Strain the leaves and zest out of the oil and pour the oil into a sterilized bottle. Use within 2 months.

Another mosquito repellent

Mugwort (*Artemisia vulgaris*) was used in many ways by the ancient Slavs and was considered one of their most magical herbs. It seems to grow absolutely everywhere in Europe (and beyond too, I expect).

MAKES 1 BUNCH

1 sprig of mugwort
20cm (8in) piece of natural string (optional)

◎ Place the mugwort in a sunny spot to dry out for a couple of hours.

◎ Take the shorter stalks off the main stem and create a bunch with the stalks roughly the same length. If you have string, tie it from one end to the other. If you don't, you can burn the branches individually.

◎ Light the bunch of mugwort, placing it in a ceramic pot when not holding it.

THE MYTH OF *POŁUDNICA*

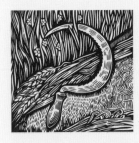

It was harvest time. She came in the heat of the midday sun in a cloud of dusty haze, carrying a sharp silver sickle in her thin hand. She wore a wreath of wheat about her head and wispy, white cloths over her bones. Her victims might faint, suffer burns, get a migraine and become disorientated, or sometimes even die as they were attacked.

She had many names and came in a few different guises. *Południca* refers to the time of day she comes. Other names reflected the fields in which she was found. While some said she was eye-wateringly beautiful (so as to easily capture men's attention) and sang as she walked (in order to make her victims sleepy), others said she was shockingly thin and very old or looked like the undead. In the east there was a belief that she had iron teeth.

It was said that people angered her, as they made too much noise, especially grown men and children. She never attacked a group, only stood in wait for her opportunity. The victims of the *Południca* tended to be men and often drunk men, unsurprisingly perhaps, or ones that were over-worked or ill. *Południce* were also known to be particularly cruel to children.

I heard one story of when a *Południca* kidnapped a child. It was so incredibly hot, that when the children fell asleep, the girl looking after them (still very young herself) decided to take a dip in the river. As soon as the evil spirit saw an opportunity, she stole the sleeping toddler away. When the girl came back, she was beside herself with worry. She followed the sound of soft, eerie singing to the edge of the wheat field and courageously won the child back by making up tricky riddles for the *Południca*.

The warning sign that a *Południca* was coming was a hot, dusty wind that began on an otherwise clear day. This is when the smart field peasants immediately stopped harvesting and went inside.

The belief was that *Południca* were women who died young, engaged but never married, though in ancient times, they may have been goddesses who took care of the fields rather than attacking unsuspecting peasants. The function of the *Południca* is clear: she dissuaded many an overkeen worker from the fields at midday and ensured that children stayed away from the midday sun.

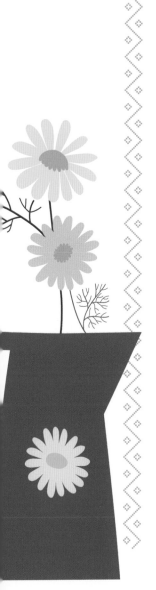

COOLING CHAMOMILE ICED TEA for a calm, summer afternoon

Summer's hot weather can bring about all kinds of frustrations and difficulties. As the myth of the *Południce* clearly shows, this is not a new issue, but has been in the human consciousness since ancient times. A cooling chamomile tea drunk in the shade of a large tree is the perfect refreshment for such a hot day and has the added benefit of making you feel calm and collected.

Sunny white and yellow chamomile (*Matricaria chamomilla*) appears to grow everywhere in the summer, but the fact is that many other wildflowers look just like it. Usually, you can tell chamomile apart from the rest by its wispy dill-like leaves, but then there is fake chamomile, which also has those, yet no scent.

Chamomile is common, and its lookalikes don't tend to be poisonous, but make sure, as always, that you know exactly what you are picking. Chamomile is reputed to be best in early summer, when picked on a warm dry day, at about midday.

If you want to take the tea to a picnic, then simply pop it into a thermos flask to keep cool.

SERVES 4

Large bunch of fresh chamomile flowers (about 100g/3½oz)
3 tablespoons good-quality honey
1l/35fl oz/4¼ cups warm water from a pre-boiled kettle
Juice of ½ lemon

◉ Allow the chamomile flowers to rest in the sun for 20 minutes, so that any bugs can leave, then rinse under cold running water.

◉ Place the flowers in a jug, add the honey and pour over the warm (not hot) water. Cover and allow to cool to room temperature.

◉ Add the lemon juice, then serve over ice, or keep in the refrigerator for later.

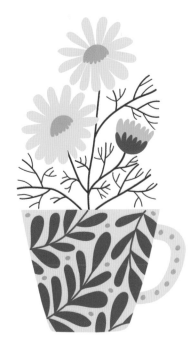

WILD SALAD for a magical midsummer meal

This wild salad can be adapted to your own environment and needs. I've suggested the kind of wild greens you can use during the summer.

Dandelion greens can be found everywhere, and their taste is not a million miles from rocket/arugula. Their benefits include lowering inflammation and blood pressure, among other things.

The name "pigweed" doesn't sound lovely in English, yet this common weed has been used by Slavs for generations. In Poland, it brings to mind poverty; people used to eat it because they had to. Yet it turns out that it has many benefits, including aiding digestive health.

Mugwort was considered a magical herb by the Slavs and was used to contact the other realms by wise men and women of these lands in the past. The flowers (they look more like seeds) also happen to be delicious, especially when roasted.

SERVES 2

2 tablespoons mugwort flowers
   (*Artemisia vulgaris*)
2 handfuls of dandelion greens
   (*Taraxacum officinale*)
2 handfuls of lamb's quarters/wild
   spinach/pigweed (*Chenopodium album*)
2 tablespoons sunflower seeds
1 tablespoon cold-pressed sunflower oil
A few edible flowers, such as marigolds,
   nasturtium or cornflowers
Salt

FOR THE VINAIGRETTE
3 tablespoons cold-pressed sunflower oil
1 tablespoon lemon juice or apple cider
   vinegar (page 148)
1 teaspoon mayonnaise
½ teaspoon mild mustard
salt and white pepper

First, dry the mugwort flowers by laying them out on baking sheets lined with greaseproof/wax paper in the sunshine for 20 minutes. They should smell herbaceous and delicious already at this point.

Wash the dandelion greens and pigweed gently and allow to dry.

Place the vinaigrette ingredients in a jar and shake vigorously to combine. Shake again before using.

Add the sunflower seeds to the baking sheet with the dried mugwort and drizzle with the sunflower oil. Mix together with your hands so everything is evenly coated, season with salt and roast for 25–30 minutes at 180°C/350°F/ Gas mark 4, stirring halfway through.

Place the dandelion greens and pigweed on your serving plate and drizzle with half the vinaigrette. Scatter over the crunchy mugwort and sunflower seeds and drizzle with the other half of the vinaigrette.

Whimsically throw the edible flowers over the top of the salad before serving it as part of your magical midsummer meal.

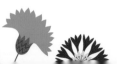

ARONIA *NALEWKA* for pleasant detoxification

The tartly bitter aronia is native to those furthermost areas where Russia almost kisses America. Nowadays, Poland is one of the largest producers of this mouth-drying superfood, fittingly called chokeberry in English. In order to reduce this effect and make the most of its many health benefits, we simply need to cook the berries. Aronia berries are known to cleanse the body of toxins, acting as an antibacterial and antifungal. This *nalewka* – vodka medicine – is used to calm the stomach, lower cholesterol and even improve the condition of hair and nails. It's an elegant *nalewka* – not too sweet – and was a favourite of my Babcia Halinka.

Note:
We pick chokeberries near the end of summer.

MAKES 1 x 2l/70fl oz JAR

700g/1lb 9oz aronia/chokeberries
350ml/12fl oz good-quality runny honey
500ml/17fl oz/2 cups vodka
Juice of ½ lemon
2l/70fl oz sterilized glass jar
2l/70fl oz sterilized glass bottle

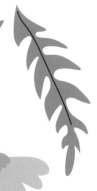

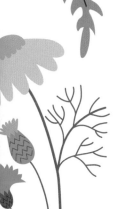

◙ Wash the berries, then allow them to dry naturally. Place them in the freezer overnight.

◙ The next day, put the berries in the jar and cover with the honey. Close the lid and leave in a warm, dark place for 2 days, stirring once a day.

◙ On the third day, add the vodka and the lemon juice. Stir, put the lid back on and leave for 4 weeks.

◙ Strain out the fruit and pour the liquid into a sterilized bottle.

◙ Allow to mature for 4–6 months, turning the bottle upside down whenever you remember.

MIRABELLE JAM
to relieve stress

There's something magical about mirabelles (*Prunus domestica subsp. syriaca*). I find it very difficult to drive past a bountiful mirabelle tree full of the bright, ripe fruit without stopping to collect some. But if you don't have time to do something with them that day (or the next day at the very latest), then you should wait, as these fruit go off very quickly. They say that the best mirabelles are the ones that have already dropped to the ground, although we clearly don't want any that are going off. The best thing to do in this case is shake the tree, so that only the ones that are ready but still fresh drop.

Mirabelles are rich in vitamin B and minerals, and therefore they help maintain good health in a myriad of ways; however, one of the most important benefits for our modern lives is that they help to relieve stress. I feel that the jam-making process has a similar effect on my stress levels.

MAKES 1 x 250ml/9fl oz JAR

600g/1lb 5oz mirabelle plums
300g/10½oz/1½ cups golden
　caster/granulated sugar
Vanilla seeds from 1 vanilla pod
　or 1 teaspoon of vanilla extract
250ml/9fl oz sterilized glass jar

◉ Wash and destone the fruit and place them in a saucepan with the sugar. Leave for at least 6 hours to release their juices.

◉ Place the pan over a low heat and cook gently for about an hour, stirring often so that nothing sticks to the bottom of the pan.

◉ Once the jam is thick and jelly-like, transfer it to the sterilized jar. Screw the lid on and turn the jar upside down, while the filling is still hot. This will seal it well.

ELDERBERRY SYRUP
in preparation for a change of seasons

We never actually planted the elderberry tree (*Sambucus nigra*) in our garden. The elderberry attached itself to another plant and we had no idea what it was. In time, it killed off (strangled, I believe) that other plant to grow into a majestic tree at the back of our garden. I have to admire its persistence. Now, I also appreciate its gifts, which the other, more decorative plant would not be offering to us. Tart black elderberries release their toxins once cooked, so that we can then benefit from their nutrients. They come at the end of summer, when your immune system could really do with a helping hand. I often miss my opportunity and forget to pick them at the right time, then kick myself when I get that annoying end-of-summer cold. Then I look wistfully upon the few elderberries still left on the trees and wonder if there are enough to make a few spoonfuls of syrup. The birds never miss an opportunity.

Note:
Some recent Norwegian studies showed that elderberry syrup can reduce the period flu symptoms are suffered by up to 4 days

MAKES 1 x 250ml/9fl oz BOTTLE

250g/9oz elderberries, rinsed
150ml/5fl oz/²/₃ cup water
120g/4oz/²/₃ cup golden caster/granulated sugar or 150ml/5fl oz/²/₃ cup good-quality honey
250ml/9fl oz sterilized glass bottle

◉ Remove the elderberries from the stems (I like to use a fork). Place them in a saucepan, cover with the water and bring to the boil.

◉ Turn the heat down and simmer for 10 minutes before turning the heat off and allowing to cool to room temperature. Strain out the plant matter and add the sugar or honey.

◉ Heat again, while stirring continuously. Do not boil. Once the sugar has dissolved, pour the still-warm syrup into the sterilized bottle. It should last for about 2 months in the refrigerator.

◉ Take a teaspoonful a day once the weather is starting to cool and you feel that autumn is coming.

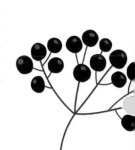

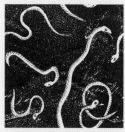

THE SNAKE

In earlier days, snakes were venerated all over the Slavic lands. A snake was considered to have supernatural powers, in part due to the shedding of its skin, which represents rebirth. It was both feared and respected. The snake symbolized a king with a crown on his head.

The Southern Slavs especially have been known to worship snakes. In Montenegro, there was a belief that a black snake lived under every house, and if it was killed, then the head of the house would die. In Slovenia, there is the myth of a *duhovin*, a child born as a snake with special abilities. In the Baltics, many families kept a harmless green snake in honour of the goddess Saule, who would reward them with prosperity and fertility.

Certain water-snakes with fiery heads were also considered of the same importance as the evil dragons (or hydra) who, at one time, threatened ships sailing on the Lake of Scutari. One of these hydras is still supposed to live in the Lake of Rikavatz, in the deserted mountains of Eastern Montenegro, from the bottom of which the hidden monster rises out of the water from time to time, and returns heralded by great peals of thunder and flashes of lightning. (Petrovitch, 1914)

In the lands that are now Poland and Ukraine, there were many stories of women marrying snakes. My favourite is a Cossack one. A peasant man meets a serpent who tells him what he needs to do for good fortune. He works as the serpent instructed, bringing in all his master's crops and asking for nothing but a sheath of corn. From this sheath springs a wonderful wife who helps bring happiness and prosperity. However, one day the peasant gets angry and calls her a serpent and, due to the man not being able to hold his tongue, she becomes a serpent. He mourns her greatly, and eventually she takes pity on him and asks him to kiss her three times. For each kiss, he is given otherworldly wisdom of how the universe works, all the languages of men and everything below the earth's surface. The serpent-wife then instructs him to go to the castle of the tsar. As a result of his great wisdom, the tsar allows him to marry his daughter.

In terms of magic, dried snake was used as a poison and shedded snake skins were the main part of a magical potion that made hair grow fast. The potion came with a warning that the hair of whoever took it could potentially wind around their neck and suffocate them, just like a snake.

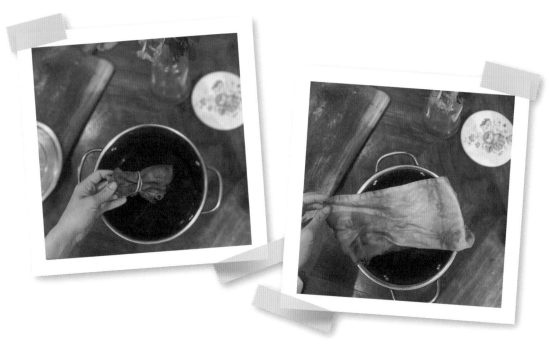

DYEING CLOTHES NATURALLY for a "new skin" - reinvention and renewal

The end of summer has always been my time for reinvention and renewal of my personal style, more so than the start of the calendar year. When I go on holiday, spending time away from my usual environment always changes me a little and so my wardrobe needs an overhaul on my return. I don't like to throw things away, so for years I used to put a bag of clothes aside for a clothes-swapping session with some friends before going to a charity shop with the remainder. I have acquired some lovely clothes this way too, from friends who actually go clothes shopping. However, my method has now changed and I lament some of the lovely fabrics I've given away.

My new method was inspired by my aunt Wiesia when I saw her in the Polish Spa town of Ciechocinek where she lives. Wiesia looked stunning in an unusual deep-coloured dress of various ethnic fabrics. When I commented on her dress, she told me that she had taken some unworn items of clothing to a *krawcowa* – seamstress – and made a new dress from them. What a brilliant idea! When I got back home, I quickly started pulling clothes out of the "to give away" bag and choosing fabrics that suited me and would go well together. That's how my new method began. I wish I could sew myself; however, I find that putting two items of clothing together is a relatively simple and cheap affair if you have a good seamstress. The satisfaction it gives you for not taking part in the disposable fashion culture is priceless.

The Wiesia method, as I like to call it, has evolved into using plants to dye some fabrics in order to either make them look more interesting, to compliment my colouring or that of the item it's being combined with, or to give it a vintage feel.

My dyeing journey began with the use of tea bags, which created an interesting effect on a frilly white cotton blouse and made it look vintage. However, my subsequent dyeing attempts were far less satisfactory. You would have thought that beetroot would make an excellent dye – not so! I had to go back and do some research.

Dyeing fabrics in Poland has been traced back to the ancient and remarkably preserved settlement of Biskupin, where lady's bedstraw and elder were used to dye garments red and blue respectively. We know knotgrass and yellow iris were used to dye both threads and garments blue and yellow in Gdańsk in the 12th and 13th centuries. The ancient Slavs were known to dye linen and wool, which were important cottage industries at the time. Since having children, I've found that I'm uncomfortable in synthetic fabrics, so I only wear breathable cotton and linen. As a rule, I only ever dye natural fabrics, as synthetics tend to repel natural dyes. I don't consider myself to be an expert, only someone who enjoys experimenting with natural dyes. Since it brings me joy, I wanted to share this ancient kitchen art with you. I love the surprise element of using natural plant matter because you never quite know what will happen, even if you have used that plant before.

There are many variables with natural dyeing. The amount of dye product is tricky to define and takes some experimentation because it depends on the intensity of colour you want, the type of natural dye you are using, the material you are dyeing and how long you simmer it for. The colour of the dye is, in addition, dependent on the time of year, the soil in the area and which part of the plant you use. Different fixers also have different effects. In the natural dyeing world, most dyers swear by alum mordant (or an aluminium stone) to fix the dye onto the fabric; iron mordant, on the other hand, drastically changes the colour of the natural dye and is loved by more experienced dyers. Although both alum and iron are found in tap water, using them in larger quantities (you need protective gear for this) is not something I feel comfortable doing in my family kitchen. I therefore only use plant materials that contain tannins, such as trees and shrubs (see below) so that I don't need use any mordant at all.

I won't hide that part of the appeal of dyeing for me is that we are imparting health-giving properties from the plant into the item. I also give my dyed materials a lemon juice rinse (just lemon juice and water) at the end, which some say helps to fix the dye. Most importantly, I like the smell and luminescent quality that lemon juice imparts on the material. I am always open to the possibility of re-dyeing the item in the future. I treat the items with care and never wash them at a temperature higher than 30°C (86°F). Nevertheless, many of them will fade or change colour over time.

This is a journey of experimentation. This is not a method if you like your items dyed perfectly or bold, even colours. I advise you to experiment a little first before committing to dying an item you like. Once I tried to recreate the look of the aforementioned frilly white blouse on an apricot cotton jumper and ended up with a dirty-looking jumper. I just dyed it again until I was happy with the colour,

so this wasn't a huge problem for me, but I enjoy being the mad professor in the kitchen and must stress that natural dyeing is not for everyone. This type of dyeing is a handmade and artisanal affair, which produces the colours of nature and an uneven finish. I like to accentuate this effect by tying plant matter up inside the fabric with an elastic band. If you would like to experiment with iron effects without adding any actual iron salts, you could tie up some rusty metal into the fabric. This can produce quite dramatic effects. While I have experimented a little with rusty objects, I stay away from both iron and alum as they are poisonous in large amounts and I usually have small children and animals in my kitchen. Personally, I enjoy combining the natural plant matter to create interesting effects and strengthen the dye (see ideas below). I also use the branches of those tannic trees to keep the fabric in place when dyeing.

If you prefer a more even dye effect then you could create the dye first. This is how to extract the dye from the plant: half fill a large pot with your natural dyeing product and cover with water (as a guide, I would say you need about twice the weight of plant product to the weight of your fabric). Leave this to stand overnight if possible, but a minimum of two hours. Bring to the boil and simmer for an hour, then add your fabrics and continue as below, without tying any plant matter into the fabric and making sure it's evenly covered during the simmering process, when air bubbles push it up.

Below are some notes on my own natural dyeing experiments.

Notes:

1. *Dedicate a very large old pot (with a lid), that you no longer want to use for cooking, for your natural dyeing experiments.*

2. *The scouring process is a great way of getting your clothes really clean. If I ever had any stained clothes in my youth, my mother would always scour them. She did it by boiling them with washing powder for an hour, but I prefer the process described on page 110.*

Dye notes:

1. *Using a fixer such as alum or iron will give (sometimes dramatically) different results.*
2. *Please be careful that you don't injure trees when using them. Prune small branches off correctly to use in dyeing.*
3. *Things that contain plenty of natural tannins include tree bark and leaves, unripe fruit, and nut shells.*

HAWTHORN – Pinks earlier in the season – bronze later in the season. Hawthorn dye can be quite variable which, for me, makes it fun to experiment with. Use large hawthorns, as the big ones won't have thorns on their branches, and, of course, we don't want to make holes in our fabric. You can easily cut a branch at the stem.

ELDER – (like the ancient inhabitants of Biskupin!) mauve, pinks, lilac. I like to use a whole branch with berries, leaves and bark. Fugitive dye turns beige over time.

BIRCH – Browns. Cut a branch with leaves at the stem and cut it further into smaller parts.

CHAMOMILE – Yellow. I like to combine this with some tannic leaves, such as birch, raspberry or elder, but I generally use about 75 per cent weight of teabags to the fabric and a few leaves and branches on top.

TEA – Beige. I achieve a rose-beige hue on white cotton by using 50 per cent teabags to the weight of fabric; darker shades require more teabags.

WALNUT SHELLS – Some say they produce **black,** but without mordant I have only achieved a **dark, chocolatey brown.**

YELLOW ONION PEELS – Yellow-beige.

RED ONION PEELS – Dusty rose pink.

CHESTNUT BARK AND LEAVES – Brown.

RED CABBAGE – Blue, violet. I use red cabbage in conjunction with tannic leaves and branches. Fugitive dye turns beige over time. Things smell of cabbage for a while.

YARROW – Light green, yellow. Ironically, it's difficult to find a green dye in nature – one with its own tannins anyway. I combine yarrow with a handful of tannic leaves/bark.

MADDER ROOT – Reds, pinks, oranges. Used for centuries to produce dyes.

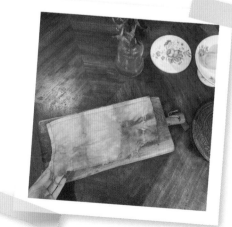

GENERAL INSTRUCTIONS

◉ First, we need to prepare the fabric by scouring it. I use 1 tablespoon of sodium carbonate (soda ash/washing soda) and 1 tablespoon of pH-neutral soap (gentle dish soap does the trick) to 3l/100fl oz/13 cups of water and bring it to the boil. Simmer for at least an hour for cotton and linen, prodding fabric down with the back of wooden spoon regularly. Rinse until the water runs clear.

◉ Add the plant matter to your large dyeing pan and cover with water. Leave for a few hours or overnight.

◉ Place some plant matter inside the garment and tie it in place with an elastic band around the outside of the garment. Pop it into the water. Bring to the boil, then turn the heat down and simmer for the amount of time your fabric needs.

◉ Simmer the garments for:
– 1.5–2 hours for linen and cotton
– 30 minutes for silk
– For wool, wait for the water to cool slightly, before immersing it for 30 minutes.

◉ Allow to cool in the dye.

◉ Finish by placing your items in very cold water and rinsing them

until the water runs clear, usually for me this means two rinses. On the second rinse, I add 100ml/ 3½fl oz/scant ½ cup lemon juice for every litre of water and allow the items to rest in it for 20 minutes. Wring the fabric out and allow it to dry naturally.

Note:

Sodium carbonate is not called soda ash for no reason. You can make it by spreading bicarbonate of soda/ baking soda on a baking sheet and putting it in the oven at 100ºC/200ºF/ Gas mark ½ for an hour.

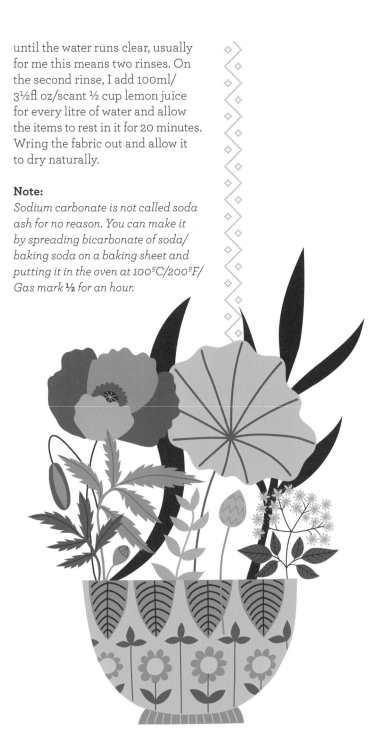

BIRCH AND HAWTHORN-DYED TROUSERS for healthy skin and lazy lounging

One of the things I love most about natural dyeing is that the plant imparts its qualities into the fabric. Not only do you get a luminescent colour that reflects the light in a magical way, you also gain benefits from the plant. Birch and hawthorn both have many health benefits and therefore by using them to dye items that are close to the skin, such as these cheap cotton-linen trousers I had, you are imparting some of their goodness through your largest organ – the skin. And, of course, you create a unique piece of clothing, like these trousers, which I like to wear around the house or even sleep in. You could also use this method to dye a bedsheet that perhaps has some stains on it. While a tablecloth won't be close to your skin, it would also look very interesting with this kind of effect.

40–50cm (16–20in) branch of both hawthorn
    and elder
Light linen/cotton trousers
Piece of string or 2 elastic bands

◙ Cut a branch of birch and branch of hawthorn off at the stem. Hawthorns, as the name suggest, can be thorny, so I would recommend that you find a hawthorn tree rather than a bush, as the large branches on the trees don't tend to have any thorns.

◙ Chop the birch branch into many smaller pieces. Place it in the pan and cover with the water. Leave to stand overnight.

◙ Scour your trousers as described opposite.

◙ Place some of the birch bark and leaves inside the still wet trousers and tie with plain elastic bands. Pop this in the pot with the birch plant material and bring the water to the boil.

◙ Simmer for about an hour, then turn the heat off and allow the garment to cool in the dye.

◙ Place the trousers in a cold-water bath and untie the plant material. Leave in the water for 5 minutes to rinse off the excess dye. Squeeze the water out (it should be running clear).

◙ Prepare a lemon water bath (as described opposite) and place your item in it for 20–30 minutes.

◙ Prepare the hawthorn dye in the same way as the birch dye, then tie up some of the plant material inside your item and place it inside the dye. Bring this to the boil and simmer for an hour, as before. Turn the heat off and allow the trousers to cool in the dye.

◙ Rinse the item in the same way as above and allow to dry naturally.

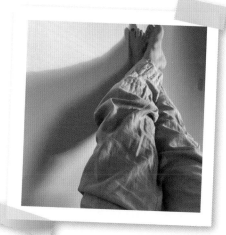

CHAMOMILE AND ELDER PILLOWCASES for a good night's sleep

Chamomile is one of the herbs I would find it very difficult to live without. The smell of it makes me feel at home. Therefore, for me, this is the ideal fragrance to use to dye personal items such as pillowcases, which I rest my face on night after night. This calming herb not only helps us to get a good night's rest, but also gives new life to some old pillowcases.

Don't forget to thank the magical elder tree when you take its branch (and cut it in the appropriate place where it's thicker too). The elder provides some more tannins to make this dye last, although, as with all the natural dyes that I use with no alum (or any other fixer, for that matter), you should be open to re-dyeing it in the future and layering on that plant colour and effect. I only ever wash these on a short wash at 30°C (86°F) in the meantime.

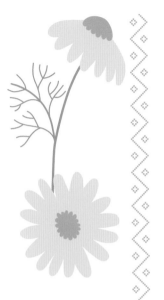

MAKES 1 PILLOW

2 white or cream pillowcases
80g/2¾oz dried chamomile flowers (see page 42, or use tea bags)
2 thin branches of elder with leaves
2 elastic bands or pieces of string

◎ Scour the pillowcases (see page 110) for at least an hour.

◎ Place the chamomile in your dyeing pan and cover with at least 2l/70fl oz/8½ cups of water. Bring to the boil, then turn the heat down.

◎ Using the back end of a wooden spoon, place the pillowcases in the chamomile dye, pushing them underneath the surface. Place the elder branches on top to keep the material in place (you'll probably have to break them in two to make them fit).

◎ Simmer together for at least an hour, prodding the air bubbles down with the back end of the wooden spoon from time to time. Allow to cool in the dye bath.

◎ Rinse well with cold water and use lemon juice with the second or final rinse (the juice of half a lemon should do it). Leave it in the lemon solution for 20 minutes, then squeeze dry and allow to dry naturally.

THE BAKER AND THE BEE (A Polish story)

Long ago, in the beautiful Polish town of Toruń, there lived a hardworking and kind baker called Bartomiej who was madly in love with a lady called Rose. As Bartomiej walked to work, he would pick wild flowers for Rose; at work, he would bake little treats especially for her. However, Rose's parents were rich, so they wanted to marry Rose off to a grumpy but wealthy old man, who could provide their daughter with everything her heart desired. What they didn't know is that Rose's heart did not care for material things and she was deeply in love with the young baker.

One pleasant summer evening, Bartomiej was walking cheerfully home from work when he felt a strong urge to go into the woods and pick some forget-me-nots for Rose. He walked off the path and into the forest. The birds were singing evening songs and the sun was still shining its warm golden glow through the tree branches. The baker walked until he reached a small clearing filled with bright wild flowers. He found a patch of forget-me-nots growing by a tiny pond and knelt down to pick them. When he looked into the pond, he noticed a bee struggling for its life, so the kind baker picked up a leaf and fished the drowning bee out of the water. He placed it on some grass to dry its wings in the sun's final warm rays and got on with picking his flowers.

All of a sudden, Bartomiej felt like he was being watched. He turned around slowly to see a bright, shiny figure perched upon a tree branch. His jaw dropped. He could not believe his eyes, yet he knew instinctively who it was sitting there, because his grandma had told him many folk tales in his childhood. Sitting on an ancient linden tree was the queen of the krasnoludki pixies! She was small, perhaps the size of a cat, and there was a golden glow all around her. She smiled gently and her voice sounded like bells ringing.

"Thank you kind Bartomiej for you have saved the queen of an important clan of bees. She will go on to have many children and the clan will continue for years to come. As a token of my gratitude, I will tell you a secret that will make you your fortune. The bees have made a nest in that pine tree over there... take the honey from it and add it to your gingerbread. The bees won't hurt you..."

Bartomiej turned around to look at the tree that the queen was pointing at and when he turned back, she was gone, the branch she had sat on still swinging. The baker trusted the queen and so did as he was told. He found some bark and went over to the tree to gather honey. He was nervous putting his hand into the hive, but the bees allowed him to take all the handfuls he needed to fill the bark.

The next morning Bartomiej got up before dawn as usual and went to his work. He added the special forest honey to the gingerbread dough as he had been instructed, rolled it out and made his biscuits as usual. When he put them on to bake, their divine smell filled the bakery and wafted down the road. By the time it came to open the bakery, there was already a long queue of customers outside, all remarking on the incredible smell of gingerbread.

Soon, word got around and the whole town was in love with Bartomiej's gingerbread. The lords and ladies would request Bartomiej make huge sculptures from it for their celebrations and even the King of Poland turned to Bartomiej when there was a royal feast taking place, for his gingerbread was known to be the best in the land.

Rose's parents saw how well the young baker was doing, so, finally, they softened and gave their blessing for the marriage of Rose and Bartomiej. The happy couple had a large family and the baker passed on his secret gingerbread recipe to his children, so that the Toruń gingerbread would continue to be made in the same special way for years to come. His recipe is used to this day.

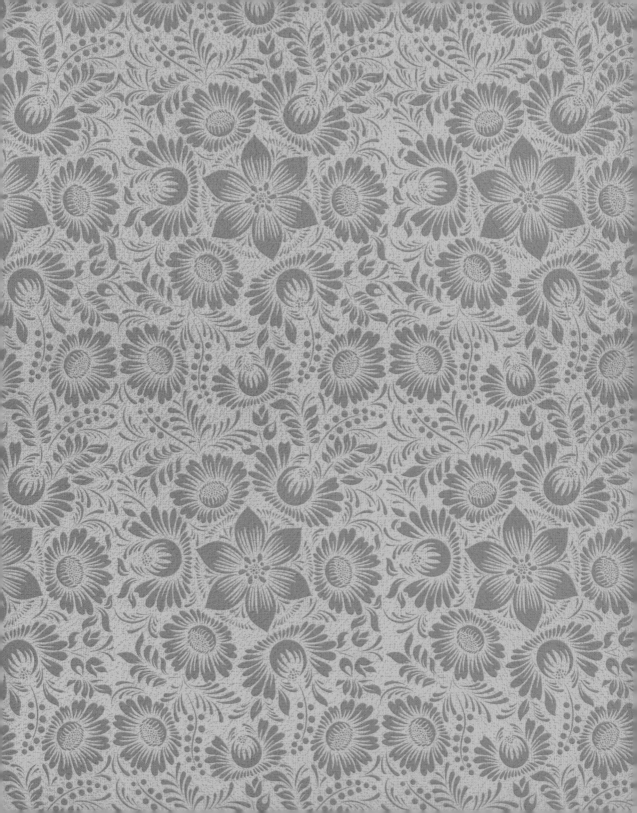

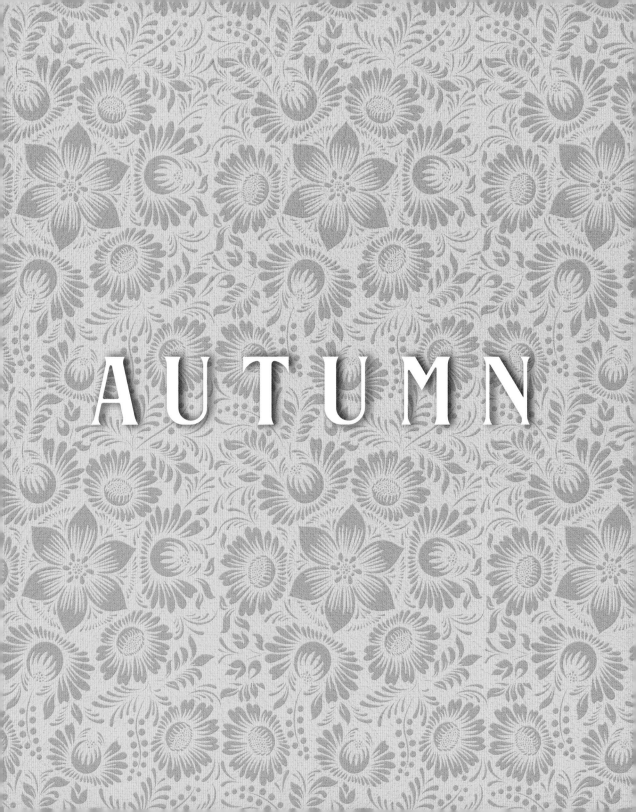

AUTUMN

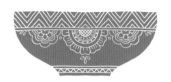

Autumn transforms; an ordinarily green tree can turn the most dazzling combination of colours as they start to let go of their life. Every leaf will need to be released and it seems that, before they go, they want to have their moment in the spotlight. Autumn is the ideal time for us to let go, too. I use this time to transform myself gently from within. I slow down, take extra time to meditate and contemplate what is and isn't working in my life. I perform rituals and pick herbs to help me take care of my health.

This is also a time of preparation. The old Slavic customs were quite specific during these months. After the harvest celebrations, it was time to start work in the kitchen. This is a busy period of preserving the harvest and preparing for a long, cold winter. We make sure that nothing goes to waste because we might need it in the coming season. While in the olden days, these kinds of preparations had the air of a military operation, our lives are easier now, so we can afford to prepare in a more relaxed manner.

Since gardens and allotments need to be cleared, this is the perfect time for bonfires, both to get rid of debris and to warm our bones after a day of outdoor work. You can also write down a list of what you are ready to let go of and pop it on the fire – an important practice to keep ourselves focused during the upcoming dark months. When a person died, all their papers used to be burnt on a fire, an old custom harking back to pagan days when the dead were burned along with the belongings they might need in the next world. To reflect the death of the earth in the approach to winter, the natural rhythm dictates that we experience something similar in our own lives. However, it does not have to be a dark or painful time because, after letting go, we will be born again into a more evolved version of ourselves. At ancient Slavic wakes, there would be feasting and dancing, a celebration of the soul's travel to a better place.

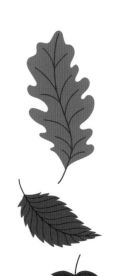

Once we are prepared for winter and the earth is beginning to fall asleep, it is a magical time when the veils between the worlds are thin. A time to connect to our ancestors. These days in Poland, we celebrate All Saints by walking around the cemeteries where our predecessors are buried. We clean the graves, light candles and bring flowers. The cemeteries smell of wax, smoke and cut flowers. It is an opportunity to see our distant family members and old friends, who will be doing the same thing. It is a time to connect, both to this world and the next.

Ci którzy bliżej cmentarza mieszkali,
Wiedzą iż upiór ten co rok się budzi,
Na dzień zaduszny mogiłę odwali
I dąży pomiędzy ludzi.

He who lives near the cemetery knows
That this ghost every year doth rise,
On All Souls' out of the grave he goes
To be among people, he strives.

(Adam Mickiewicz, *Dziady*, trans. Zuza Zak)

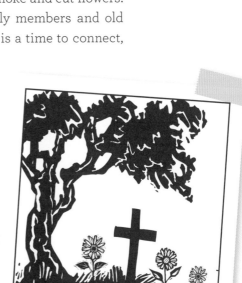

Before Christianity, in Poland, Belarus, Ukraine and Russia, we celebrated Dziady – meaning "forefathers" – a day of Slavic folk rituals intended to achieve communion with the ancestors. Food and drink, such as *kasza* (groats or grains), were brought to the graves. It was also popular to spill some honey and vodka to share it with the spirit world. Fires were lit (now the candles) to keep the dead warm. If people felt haunted by someone, this was a time to ask them what their soul needed in order to rest. It was also a time to enjoy the presence of those we loved and lost.

Slavic folklore often talks of malevolent spirits, not to mention undead beings such as vampires and werewolves. In the gothic tale of Twardowski, a nobleman makes a deal with a powerful, evil spirit. He lives a selfish life, never gets old and bosses his demonic servant about, until eventually the spirit loses patience and wants Twardowski's soul. It tricks Twardowski into going to Rome, where he can claim it. However, as he's flying through the sky with the demon, Twardowski starts singing a hymn he sang in childhood, when he was still innocent, which causes the spirit to let him go. And so Twardowski ends up floating in the clouds, stuck between this world and the next until the Day of Judgement. We can see how Christianity has asserted itself through the folk stories, as an antidote to the human fears of the dark and the unknown. In Polish folklore, Christianity feels like a comforting balm to an often hostile world. This is how I remember my Babcias treated their faith, with love and trust in a kind, protective God.

The human life cycle involves both light and shadow, same as the earth's cycle. As darkness increases, autumn brings in augmented connection with the unseen, both other dimensions and our own shadow. There is a power in this – folk stories teach us that we must not turn away, instead remaining strong, brave and resolute.

SIMPLE CANDLES for rituals, meditation and contemplation

Although candle magic has grown in popularity in recent years, I don't cast magical spells with candles. Instead, I love to use them in meditation, contemplation and in simple rituals that bring me closer to my ancestors. This has always been my instinct and whenever I am in a Catholic church, I will light candles for my loved ones that have passed.

The act of making your own candle imparts your energy into it, making it ideal for rituals. If you want to do magical spells, then please do some research first. While I'm not an expert on folk magic, I know there's a whole world of rules and regulations around folk magic. For example, I was told that you need to dispose of any candles used to heal the body within three days of the ritual, buried in the garden where no one will walk over them. Do the research if that's how you would like to use candles.

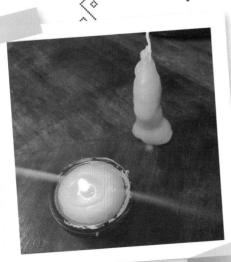

You could, if you wish, protect your candle's energy by tying a red ribbon around it when not in use. Red bows were often used as a means of protection by the Slavs, which is why they were often found on baby's cribs.

MAKES 1 RITUAL CANDLE AND 1 BEDSIDE CANDLE

130g/4½oz beeswax
1 x 20cm/8in wick
1 x 12cm/5in wick
1 tablespoon lavender essential oil
Empty, clean food can
2 metal nuts
Strong stick (I use a chopstick)
70–100ml/2½-3½fl oz sterilized glass jar
Sticky tape

◉ Place your beeswax in the can and put the can in a small saucepan. Fill the pan with 2–3cm (1in) of water, but not so much that the can floats.

◉ Set the pan over a medium heat and bring the water to the boil. Turn down the heat to low and allow all the wax to melt.

◉ Meanwhile, prepare the wicks. For the dipped ritual candle, thread one end of the longer 20cm/8in wick through a metal nut and tie a knot. Secure the other end to your stick. For the poured bedside candle, thread one end of the 12cm/5in wick through the second metal nut and tie a knot. Place it in the middle of your glass jar and secure the other end with sticky tape to the outside of the jar.

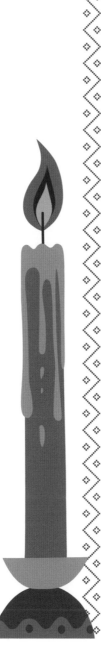

🎇 Turn the heat down under the saucepan. Dip the 20cm/8in wick in the wax, holding it by the stick. Then dip it in the water, and then the wax again. You can use an oven glove to tilt the can to the side and dip it evenly on each side.

🎇 Once you have a candle that's about 10–15cm (4–6in) tall and of a thickness you like, place it in the water.

🎇 Now, turn the heat off and stir the essential oil into the wax. Pour the rest of wax into the jar. If there is any left over, you can hold the long candle over the cold water and pour the wax over it while turning. Whatever falls into the water, you can use for some gentle divination if you like. Take a deep breath and clear your mind, then look at the shape in the water. What's the first thing you think of – this symbol will indicate something coming into your life.

🎇 For the dipped ritual candle, trim the string with the wax on it (not the weight) and the wick to about 1cm (½in). For the poured candle, trim the wick to about 1cm (½in) also.

RITUAL for honouring your ancestors

A candle ritual is one of the simplest and most beautiful ways that you can honour your ancestors, and is reputed to be especially potent at this time of year when the veil between the worlds is at its thinnest.

1 homemade candle or a simple
    beeswax candle
Matches
A photo of your ancestor/s or an
    item that belonged to them

🎇 Sit in a dark, quiet room and light your candle.

🎇 Bring to mind your ancestor/s, while holding the item that represents them. Imagine them in their happiest state. Imagine they are sitting next to you now. Send them love.

🎇 When it is time to go, thank them for being with you and blow the candle out.

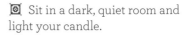

A LETTING-GO RITUAL for clarity and inner peace

I like to think of my time here on earth as a journey; every day we are moving forward in some way. When travelling, it's easiest to travel light, and to do this, it's important to let go of the things we don't need. We have so much to deal with throughout the year, so many people around us and many more on social media, all vying for our attention. People who think they know the answers and want to tell us their opinions, people who want to be seen, be believed, and have your agreement, your vote. The world is getting faster and more demanding. How do we stay calm and focused? How do we make the right decisions on a daily basis? We need to stay grounded and look inside ourselves, but in order to do that we need to quieten the world around us and focus our energy inward.

Note:
The best time to do a letting-go ritual is during the full moon.

1 homemade candle or a simple
    beeswax candle
        Pencil
        Piece of paper
        Bowl

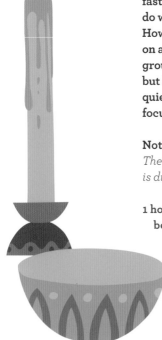

◙ Sit in a dark, quiet room and light your candle.

◙ Sit close to the candle and try to clear your mind for 5–10 minutes. If you are finding it hard to keep your mind empty and thoughts keep entering your head, that's just perfect for this exercise. Even if you are practised in meditation and letting go comes easily to you, you will no doubt still have a thought enter now and again.

◙ Focus on all the thoughts that are clinging to you. Name them, one by one. Write them down on your piece of paper. If there are negative feelings associated with your thoughts, write them down too. Each time, return to the meditation and continue to empty your mind until you have caught them all – every single thing that is bothering you. Even if it is something that isn't obviously negative, such as "I need to put the washing on", name it.

◙ Once you have your full list, read every item out loud, then finish with: "I give this list over to you [name your higher power] so that I may be free now."

◙ Light the list with the candle and place it in the bowl to burn. Blow the candle out. Sit for a moment, quietly, in the dark, and relax.

THE SLAVIC WORLD OF THE DEAD

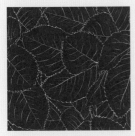 The cemeteries seem to glow on the night of All Saints' Day in Poland. As a child walking around the cemeteries for hours, the colourful candles shining upon the dark graves were constantly enticing me. I invented my own wax ritual, which included dipping my finger in as many colours of molten wax as I could fit. As each one dried, the next layer of molten wax would be applied. Eventually, a finger-shaped sculpture would emerge that I would remove from my finger, only for it to be melted back down again in the molten wax, and so on and so on ... Anything can be a meditative ritual. I have also witnessed candle wax being used for divination, either by letting candles burn out in a certain way or pouring the wax into water to see what shape it creates. Current rituals of leaving candles and flowers on graves of loved ones during All Saints' Day could point toward the ancient folk beliefs about Nawia (pronounced "Navia"), the Slavic World of the Dead. Some imagined this world to be cold and bleak, with no food, sun or beauty. Even at the beginning of last century, it was common to feast upon the graves of loved ones that have passed into this other place in order to share food with them.

Ancient Slavs believed that, after death, one soul would split into two. They thought that one part of the soul was like a human being, who could walk, sit down, eat and even breastfeed orphaned babies. This part of the soul belonged to Mother Earth and joined with the ancestors in Nawia. These are the souls that were invited to feast with us during Dziady (see page 120) and at various other times when the veils between worlds were deemed to be thin. When the spirits were around the living, people had to be careful not to step on them or bump into them (a difficult task with someone who is invisible). The other part of the soul would be reincarnated using the Tree of Life to return to its people. Depending on the type of death, some souls could also become trees, especially if they died young.

Veles, the God of the Underworld, took care of the souls in Nawia, as well as the animals of the forest. The forest and the afterlife were therefore linked. Yet, when the soul divided in two, it was said that one of the souls wanted to return to Earth. Then it was Rod (the old familial god – *rodzina* means family in Polish) and his daughters, the Rodzańce, who were given the job of taking care of the souls at the Tree of Life, until their time came to go back.

A FORTUNE-TELLING RITUAL WITH WALNUTS for an answer to your question

The Slavic people used to tell fortunes and do simple magical rituals with food items such as apples, tea, coffee and even walnuts. This is folk magic – the magic of the people – so you don't need to be guided by a magical practitioner. It is to be performed lightly and with joy. Babcia Ziuta must have mentioned the walnut divination to me because I remember wondering about it as a child. I was intrigued about how you could tell the future with walnuts, imagining that it must somehow be revealed when you open a walnut shell. My Babcia couldn't tell me, as that was not the kind of thing she partook in herself. Years later, I found this beautifully simple ritual in a book on Slavic magic – *Slavic Witchcraft* by Natasha Helvin – and the mystery was solved.

This is a fun ritual to do within a small group of close friends, and especially potent at this time of year when we know the veils between the worlds are thin. Ask everyone in your group to come up with one question they would like to have answered before you start this ritual.

FOR 1 RITUAL

13 walnuts
Piece of string about 50–60cm (20–24in) in length

◉ Make a circle on the floor from the length of string.

◉ Close your eyes for a moment and formulate your question, making sure it can be answered with a simple "yes" or "no".

◉ Say the questions aloud as you throw the walnuts into the circle.

◉ If an even number of walnuts fall within the circle, then your answer is "yes"; if it's an odd number within the circle, your answer is "no".

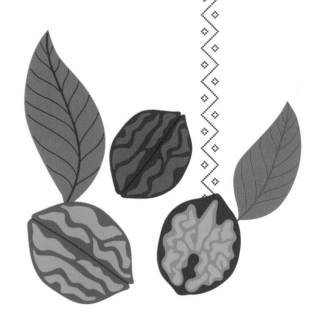

SUNFLOWER SEED *HALVA* for immunity

The Middle East has always felt close to Eastern Europe. While the Poles fought many battles against the Turks, the West often confused their Sarmatian dress with Middle Eastern garbs, viewing them as one and the same. There were also Middle Eastern communities who settled on the Slavic lands, such as the Armenians and the Tartars. All the meetings, whether friendly or bloody, brought an exchange of food and ideas. Halva has become much loved and, though usually associated with sesame seeds, I enjoy this sunflower version, which brings to mind the joyous sunflower fields of Ukraine.

MAKES 20 PIECES

300g/10½oz/2⅓ cups sunflower seeds
150g/5½oz/scant 1¼ cups plain/all-purpose flour
100g/3½oz salted butter
300ml/10½ fl oz/1¼ cups good-quality honey
1 tablespoon vanilla extract

◙ Toast the seeds in a dry frying pan until they start to colour, stirring often so they don't burn.

◙ Toast the flour in a separate frying pan, stirring continuously until it turns golden.

◙ In a food processor, blitz the seeds to a powder, reserving a few whole seeds for the top. Sift the ground seeds with the flour into a large mixing bowl.

◙ Place the butter and honey in a pan over a low heat and stir until everything has melted together. Add the vanilla, stir and turn the heat off.

◙ Combine the butter–honey mixture with the dry mixture and mix thoroughly to combine.

◙ Line a glass or ceramic dish (approx. 20cm/8in) with greaseproof/wax paper. Spoon the paste into the dish and press it down firmly.

◙ Place more greaseproof paper on top and keep pressing down for a few minutes.

◙ Scatter the remaining seeds on top and press them down into the halva, then allow to cool at room temperature before transferring to the refrigerator for at least 2 hours.

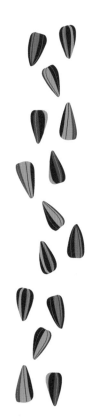

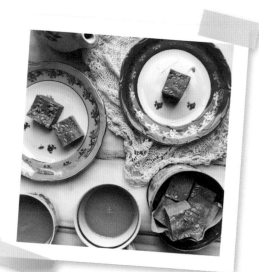

ROSEHIP INFUSION for an autumn immunity boost

Shiny red rosehips (*Rosa canina*) glowing in the sunshine tell us that autumn is here. I once heard that you should wait until after the first frost to pick the fruit, and I've also heard the exact opposite. One of the issues with folk healing is that advice can often contradict itself.

I tend to pick rosehips as soon as I get the opportunity, and, as I don't want to pick too much from one bush, I will pick over the course of a week or two, keeping them in the freezer in the meantime. I realise that some would advise against this, as it might destroy some of their nutrients, but I personally believe storage in the freezer preserves those important vitamins and minerals. I tend to pick the small rosehips, as they don't have as many hairs.

I would recommend you dry your rosehip so that you can benefit from these amazing fruits throughout the winter months – they contain more vitamin C than citrus fruit, even once dried! This is a drink I use when I feel myself starting to get ill. You can drink it for 3–4 days in a row in order to fight off that pesky cold. As rosehip contains so much vitamin C, you shouldn't drink it every day.

SERVES 1

5 fresh rosehips or 10 dried
350ml/12fl oz/1⅓ cups hot water
    from a pre-boiled kettle
1 teaspoon good-quality honey
Thermos flask

◉ If you're using fresh rosehips, wash them and remove any hairs.

◉ Place your rosehips in a thermos flask. Pour over the hot water, close the lid and allow to infuse for 5–6 hours.

◉ Strain the rosehip infusion, mix with the honey and pour it back into the flask to keep warm.

◉ Drink throughout the day (three times a day ideally).

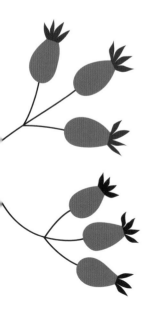

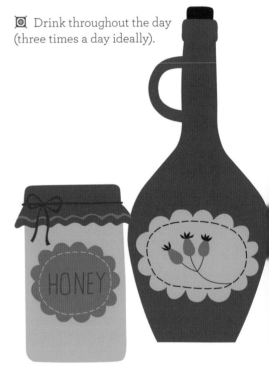

HONEY

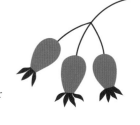

ROSEHIP *NALEWKA* for a supreme immunity boost

A rather pleasant way to boost your immunity is to take half a shot of this rosehip *nalewka* – vodka medicine – every day throughout the autumn and winter months. However, a *nalewka* needs time to age to reach its full potential (like us all) and so you will need to wait at least 3 months. The longer you leave it to mature, the better it is, so you could certainly leave at least some of it until next autumn, when you start preparing the next batch.

I collect rosehips in early autumn and freeze them until I have enough for a *nalewka*. If you don't want to freeze the rosehips, then use a knife to prick each one and let the juices come out instead.

MAKES 20 SERVINGS

120g/4½oz rosehips
250ml/9fl oz/1 cup vodka
6 tablespoons good-quality
    runny honey
250ml/9fl oz sterilized glass
    jar or bottle

◙ Place the rosehips in the sterilized jar or bottle and pour over the vodka.

◙ Leave at room temperature for 3–4 weeks, turning once a day or whenever you remember.

◙ Strain the rosehips out of the vodka, squeezing as much juice out of them as possible, then pour the vodka back into the jar or bottle.

◙ Add the honey, close the lid and shake it.

◙ Leave the *nalewka* to mature for a minimum of 3 months, turning once a day, or whenever you remember.

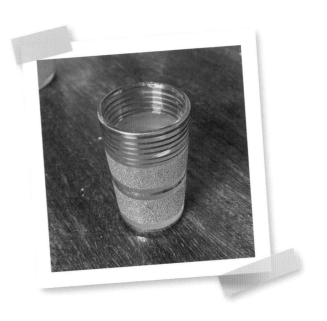

DARK RYE SOURDOUGH BREAD
with seeds and fruit for a healthy gut

Who doesn't love the smell of fresh bread wafting from the oven? It's enough to convince you to bake your own when the nights start drawing in ...

Rye is the simplest bread you can bake; it doesn't even require any kneading, as the dough is quite wet and it's meant to be a dense consistency. The dried fruit and seeds not only add to the bread's flavour and texture, but also do wonders to keep our gut healthy, strengthening our immunity at a time of the year when it's bound to be tested.

Rye has been a staple in northern Eastern Europe since the 2nd century, a miracle crop that's resistant to both the cold and pests. It also gives us strength in the form of vitamins and minerals and makes our hearts happy. While I love a crusty white loaf as much as any other bread lover, dark rye will always be my number one.

Note:
I use malt flour to improve the texture and flavour of a rye loaf. However, if you are not a regular baker and don't want to buy this ingredient, you could also use unsweetened cacao powder to a similar effect.

MAKES 1 LOAF

FOR THE STARTER
3 tablespoons wholewheat rye flour, plus 1 tablespoon for feeding
50ml/1¾fl oz warm water from a pre-boiled kettle, plus 2 tablespoon for feeding
250ml/9fl oz sterilized glass jar

FOR THE DOUGH
300g/10½oz/2½ cups wholemeal rye flour, plus extra for dusting
1 tablespoon red, barley or rye malt flour
1 teaspoon salt
2 tablespoons rolled oats
600ml/20fl oz/2½ cups warm water from a pre-boiled kettle
10 prunes, stoned and roughly chopped
2 tablespoons dried wild cherries or cranberries
2 tablespoons sunflower seeds, broken up into bits
2 tablespoons pumpkin seeds, broken up into bits
1 tablespoon cold-pressed rapeseed/canola oil

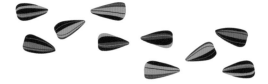

◙ To make the starter, place the rye flour and warm water in the sterilized jar and stir well with a wooden spoon to combine. Cover with a clean dish towel and leave in a warm place for 3 days, stirring once a day with a wooden spoon.

◙ On the third day, add 1 tablespoon of flour and 2 tablespoons of warm water. Stir again and leave overnight.

◙ On the fourth day, it's time to make our bread: place the rye and malt flours, salt and oats in a large bowl and mix with a wooden spoon to combine.

◙ Add some of the warm water into the jar with the starter, mix well to combine and pour into the bowl with the dry ingredients. Pour some more warm water into the jar, close the lid and shake it to collect any leftover starter remaining in the jar. Add that to the large bowl as well. Pour the rest of the warm water straight in and mix vigorously for a few minutes with a wooden spoon.

◙ After about 3–4 minutes, remove 2 tablespoons of the mixture for your next starter. Place this back in the (rinsed) jar. Once it's at room temperature, you can place it in the fridge. It will keep for a couple of weeks, but ideally use it after one week. Wake it up by adding ½ tablespoon of flour and 1 tablespoon of water, mixing well and leaving at room temperature overnight.

◙ Now add the dried fruit and seeds to the dough and mix well to combine.

◙ Grease a 900g/2lb loaf tin with the oil, then dust it with rye flour. Turn the dough out into the tin, cover with a clean dish towel and leave to rise overnight (10–12 hours) in a warm place.

◙ Preheat the oven to 180°C/ 350°F/Gas mark 4.

◙ Bake the bread for 1 hour – when it's done it should sound hollow when tapped.

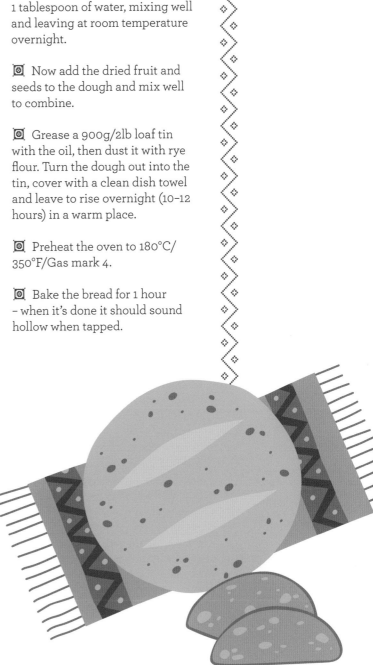

DRIED APPLES AND PEARS to aid digestion

Apples were used in many old Slavic magic rituals. They could be used to attract your love and even remove bad luck. One of the most simple and satisfying rituals I have come across asks you to imagine all your worries being transferred into an apple. Then you cut the apple in four and bury the quarters away from one another, saying goodbye to worries as you do so (Natasha Helvin talks about this in *Slavic Witchcraft*). Dried apples were some of the first Christmas decorations too, before colourful paper came along.

Drying fruit and vegetables is the oldest method of preservation. It's an incredibly practical method too, being cheap, easy and without need for bottles or jars. Through dehydration, 1kg/2lb 4oz of fresh fruit and vegetables turns into about 100–150g/3½–5½oz of dried product. Unfortunately, the dried product loses not only water but also vitamins. However, even in their dried form they are still beneficial for digestion. They can be used to create delicious, healthy snacks and they have an aromatic flavour that we can add to our recipes. I particularly enjoy the flavour of dried fruit such as apples and pears. We can either dry these fruits outside, in the sunshine if the weather is stable, or indoors at a low temperature in our ovens, in a regulated environment.

The traditional method of sun-drying was to use a big sieve and lay a thin layer of clean straw over it, place the fruit on this, a gauze over the top to protect it from dust, and finally the whole thing was placed on a sunny roof. However, I don't recommend anyone to start climbing onto their roof. You could place your fruit and vegetables on the roof of a shed or outhouse if you don't have lots of foxes and squirrels where you live (they would surely be able to make a hole in the gauze!). Otherwise, just find the sunniest spot you can for sun-drying.

If there's a lot of moisture in the air, then it's best to dry your fruit in an oven. Place the fruit and vegetable slices (not touching one another) on baking sheets lined with greaseproof/wax paper, and dry in the oven at 60°C/140°F for 30 minutes, before reducing the temperature to 50°C/120°F for a further 2½ hours. If you don't have a fan oven, then you need to open the oven and let air in at regular intervals (for example, every 30 minutes for 5 minutes).

My Babcia Ziuta also dried fruit on top of a radiator, under a clean dish towel. Another old method of drying apples was to thread the apple circles onto a bit of string and hang next to a warm hearth.

Apples

You need apples that are fresh and healthy looking, no bruises or discolourations.

◎ Whatever drying method you choose, firstly, wash and pat the apples dry. Take out the central cores and cut the unpeeled fruit horizontally into slices no thicker than 5mm (¼in).

◎ Blanch the apple slices in boiling water with lemon juice (2 tablespoons lemon juice to 1l/35fl oz/4¼ cups water) for 1 minute, then remove with a slotted spoon and drain on some paper towels. Blot dry gently, then transfer to your drying apparatus of choice.

◎ I like to dust my apples with cinnamon before drying.

◎ See the recipe introduction for drying techniques.

Pears

You need pears that are flavourful and at the perfect moment of ripeness – not too hard, not too soft. Grab them when they're just starting to become softer.

◎ Whatever drying method you choose, firstly, wash and pat the pears dry, then take out the central cores and cut the unpeeled fruit into slices no thicker than 5mm (¼in).

◎ Blanch the pear slices in boiling water with lemon juice (2 tablespoons lemon juice to 1l/35fl oz/4¼ cups water) for 1 minute, then remove with a slotted spoon and drain on some paper towels. Blot dry gently, then transfer to your drying apparatus of choice.

◎ I like to dust my pears with cardamom before drying.

◎ See the recipe introduction for drying techniques.

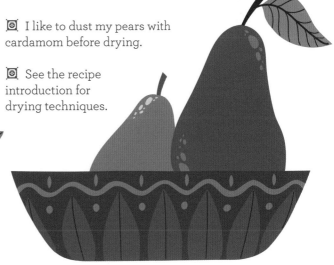

HAWTHORN BERRY AND AUTUMN FRUIT *KOMPOT* for ageing gracefully

The magical hawthorn berry (*Crataegus monogyna*), often left for the birds, is one of our secret tools for happy, healthy ageing. I find our society's obsession with stopping ageing rather odd because it's the most natural thing in the world. Nevertheless, I believe that we would all like to age gracefully and healthily. We want our skin to feel radiant and our body supple and strong.

Hawthorn has so many health benefits. It's often used to strengthen the hearts of the elderly, but I think we should start using it far earlier to reap the full benefits of this common shrub (once you know it, you'll see it everywhere!). The berries are full of vitamin C and antioxidants. They don't have a huge amount of flavour, so I like to combine them with apples and pears in this autumnal Polish drink. *Kompot* is a homemade lightly sweet drink made from any fruit, which can be consumed both warm or cold – I personally recommend warm at this time of the year.

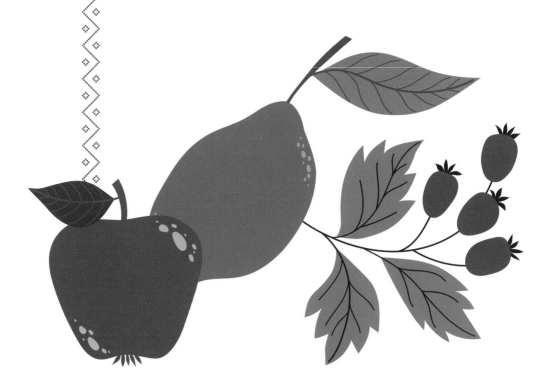

If you have stores of dried apples or pears and hawthorn berries, you can make this drink throughout winter too in order to boost your immunity and make you feel radiant. If you would like to do this, then you will need 100g/3½oz dried apples and 50g/1¾oz both dried hawthorn berries and dried pears. Cook everything together.

To dry:

Arrange the washed and air-dried berries on a baking sheet lined with greaseproof/wax paper, so that they don't touch. Place in a warm but turned-off oven at about 50°C/120°F for 3 hours or on a warm radiator, covered with a dish towel, for a day.

SERVES 4-5

150g/5½oz hawthorn berries
300g/10½oz apples
150g/5½oz pears
1.5l/52fl oz/6½ cups water
100g/3½oz/½ cup unrefined sugar
1 cinnamon stick

◙ Wash the hawthorn berries, apples and pears.

◙ Chop the apples and pears into small chunks, taking the cores out at the same time (but don't peel them). Place in one saucepan and put the hawthorn berries in another saucepan.

◙ Cover the hawthorn berries with 4 tablespoons of the water and 2 tablespoons of the sugar and cook until they disintegrate. This should take about 5 minutes.

◙ Cover the apples and pears with the remaining water and bring to the boil. Turn the heat down, then add the cinnamon stick and the rest of the sugar. Simmer for 7–8 minutes.

◙ When the apples and pears have finished cooking, turn the heat off and add the hawthorn berry mixture. Cover and allow to cool to warm.

◙ Strain the fruit out of the *kompot* but place a few apple bits into the jug or bottom of each glass (*kompot* is always served in glasses).

◙ Serve while still a little warm.

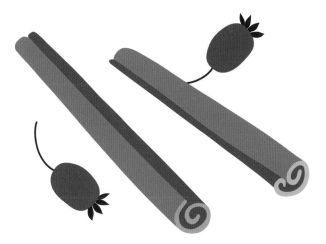

KRASNOLUDKI and other helpful daemons

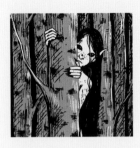

Krasnoludki are usually depicted as helpful forest-dwelling gnomes in Polish fairy tales and songs, who use mushrooms as their shelter and play pranks on people. In the old Polish tradition, which also applies to parts of Ukraine and Lithuania, *krasnoludki* – or *kraśniaki*, as they were often called in folk stories – were helpful protective spirits. Each household was thought to have a house spirit, unless it had been offended and left at some point. In the areas that are now Poland, it was often envisioned as a *krasoludek*, who lived in a little mouse hole or barn and was given scraps of food left over from dinner each night in order to keep it satisfied (when angered, the house spirit could also cause mischief). The word *krasne* suggests beauty, light and the colour red, whilst *ludek* means "little person".

Some envisioned the house spirits differently. The southern Slavs had the aforementioned house snake (see page 104), but even in what's now Poland, many differences existed between the regions. The names varied even between neighbouring villages. Some referred to the house spirit as *dziadek* – grandad – bringing to mind a kind, old man who likes to sleep on top of the stove (as old people tended to in the olden days). In and around Belarus, the name *domowik*, deriving from *dom* – house – was popular. Some even called this friendly spirit the "house devil" – *diabeł domowy* – which clearly makes it seem more severe. The *krasnoludki* (or *skrzaty* as they were also known) were imagined to shapeshift into chickens or geese.

In time came Christianity, and many of the smaller deities, such as the house spirits, were sadly (and literally) demonized. However, they were so ingrained in the Slavic psyche that their protective role needed to be filled with something, which is where the Angel Gabriel came in. While I was growing up, and for centuries prior, many children would have a picture of the angel looking after children, hanging near their bed at home – even when, like my family, theirs wasn't a particularly religious household. Even now, when my daughter is scared, I say the prayer to Angel Gabriel that I was taught by my Babcias. While I am not a practising Catholic, this protective prayer holds power for me, as it calls forth the protective energy that I know is there and always has been.

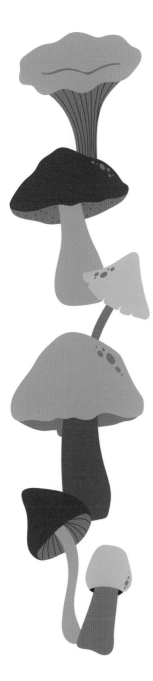

ŁAZANKI WITH WILD MUSHROOMS AND SAUERKRAUT for strong bones

Łazanki are the most rustic of all Polish pastas, even though they are said to be a relative of lasagna that came east during the 16th century. They are just boiled – sometimes fried – squares of thin dough. Everyone remembers *łazanki* from their childhoods, but hardly anyone makes them any more, though they used to be very popular in Poland, Lithuania and Belarus. I love them for their versatility. You can use them in both sweet and savoury dishes, so make extra and keep them in your refrigerator for quick mid-week meals.

Mushrooms are one of the few food sources of vitamin D. However, you need to be careful if you're foraging for them – make sure you know what you're picking, and if not, use caution. Mushrooms are a vital addition to our meals as the days start to draw in and it's difficult to get enough vitamin D from sunlight alone. In order to increase the vitamin D in your mushrooms, simply clean them, lay them out on a baking sheet lined with paper towels and allow them to sunbathe in your garden or on a sunny windowsill (with the window open) for around 30–40 minutes. Mushroom pickers tend to do this instinctively so that

the bugs can leave, but it has the added benefit of creating this important vitamin. Vitamin D has many roles in the body, one of them helping your body to absorb calcium.

While Slavs have fermented many foods over the centuries as a method of survival in the winter, sauerkraut has become perhaps the most popular one. The brine itself is considered a cure-all (for hangovers and colds alike). If you buy sauerkraut, then make sure it has no preservatives.

SERVES 4

FOR THE DOUGH
100g/3½oz/¾ cup light rye flour
100g/3½oz/¾ cup plain/
    all-purpose flour, plus extra for
    dusting
2 large pinches of salt
2 tablespoons cold-pressed
    rapeseed/canola oil
100ml/3½fl oz/scant ½ cup warm
    water from a pre-boiled kettle

FOR THE SAUCE
300g/10½oz mixed wild mushrooms
2 tablespoons cold-pressed
    rapeseed/canola oil
1 small onion or 2 shallots, finely
    chopped
200g/7oz sauerkraut, drained and
    roughly chopped
1 teaspoon finely chopped fresh
    lovage or thyme
1 tablespoon butter (salted
    or unsalted)

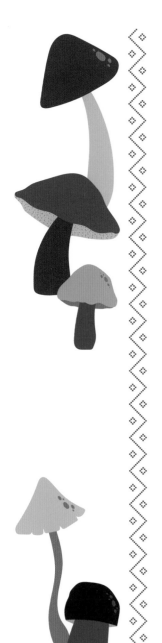

Splash of beer/apple juice/apple
  cider vinegar and water
Salt and white pepper

TO SERVE
Soured cream
More fresh lovage or thyme (optional)

◙ Place the flours for the dough in a large bowl. Add the salt, and drizzle in the oil with one hand, while rubbing it into the flour with the other. Add the water slowly, and bring the dough together. As soon as it comes together, stop adding water. Bring it into a ball, then place on a floured surface and knead for 6–7 minutes, incorporating any flour you need until the dough is smooth and elastic. Cover with a damp dish towel and allow to rest for 15–20 minutes.

◙ Meanwhile, make the sauce. First, clean your wild mushrooms. If you are using something like chanterelles, then I find it best to clean them in a sink full of water, using a small knife to scrape away any stubborn dirt. Other mushrooms may just need a rinse under running water and a light scrub with your fingers.

◙ Chop the mushrooms to roughly the same size, then pat dry with paper towels.

◙ Bring a large saucepan of water to the boil and add ½ teaspoon salt.

◙ Heat the oil in a frying pan, add the onions or shallots and fry until golden – about 5 minutes. Remove the onions/shallots from the pan.

◙ Add the wild mushrooms and fry until golden, in batches if your frying pan isn't big enough.

◙ Add the sauerkraut, fried onions/shallots and herbs to the now golden mushrooms and fry for a couple of minutes, stirring often.

◙ Add the splash of beer/apple juice/apple cider vinegar. Season with salt and white pepper. Turn the heat down and allow to cook for a further 5 minutes, stirring occasionally.

◙ Sprinkle a work surface with flour and roll the dough out as thin as you can get it (about 5mm/¼in thick). Use a sharp knife to cut the dough vertically into strips about 4–5cm/2in thick, then cut horizontally so that you end up with lots of pasta squares.

◙ In a clean frying pan, melt half the butter, then turn the heat off.

◙ Boil the *łazanki* in the salted water in batches. When you place them in the water, stir so that they don't stick to the bottom. When they float to the top, give them 2–3 minutes more, then remove with a slotted spoon, shaking off excess water, and pop them into the pan with the melted butter.

◉ Turn the heat on under the frying pan and fry the *łazanki* for 2 minutes on each side, then place them in the pan with the sauce. Repeat until you have fried all the *łazanki*, adding more butter when necessary.

◉ Heat the *łazanki* and the sauce together gently, stirring regularly – about 5 minutes should suffice.

◉ Serve with sour cream and more fresh herbs on top, if you like.

To make your own sauerkraut:

½ **small cabbage**
1 **tablespoon sea salt**
For a 500g/18oz sterilized jar

◉ Chop the cabbage finely, place in a ceramic bowl and sprinkle with the salt. Rub the salt in with your hands, then pound the cabbage gently until it starts to release some juice. Place a plate over the bowl and leave for 24 hours, pressing the plate down every hour, or whenever you remember.

◉ After 24 hours, transfer the cabbage to the sterilized jar, pressing it down every time you add a new layer. If by the time you

fill the jar and press the cabbage down, there is enough juice to cover the cabbage, then add a clean weight on top, to make sure it's fully submerged, and leave for a further 2–3 days with the lid loosely on. If there is not enough juice, then add tepid salted water to the jar, to make sure the cabbage is submerged, then add the weight etc.

◉ After 2–3 days, smell the cabbage; it should smell pleasant. Taste it and if you like it, screw the lid on and place it in the refrigerator. If you would prefer it more fermented, then let it stand for a further 24 hours, before putting it in the refrigerator. There shouldn't be any mould; if there is, even though some may be innocuous, I would recommend that you start again using a clean bowl and another sterilized jar.

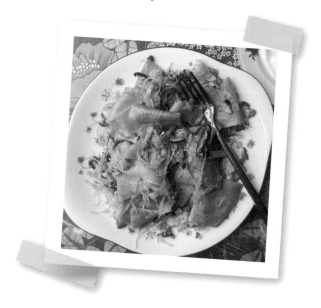

THE RAVEN

In many folk tales from the Christianized Slavic world, ravens are seen as bad omens, bringing news of death and misfortune, signifying evil witches and dark magic. The mythical Black Book of sorcery is said to be lost to humans, yet known to ravens, whilst the ancient art of Ravenplay, or divination by looking at the flight of birds, was banned by the Church along with astrology.

However, to the ancient Slavs, a raven was a respected messenger. They believed that ravens were chosen by the gods to relay both messages and souls, and fulfilled the most crucial function of bringing souls between this world and the next. While the raven carried out its duties during the dark autumn and winter months, the stork, who had similar work (and is still associated with birth) carried them out during the spring and summer.

There is an ancient Polish folk saying that goes *Kruk krukowi oka nie wykole*; translated, it means "a raven won't take another raven's eye out". As this folk saying shows, the Slavic ancestors respected ravens for being able to work together, rather than fight one another. We can't help but compare them unfavourably to men in this case. Ravens and crows often followed groups of soldiers going to battle, waiting for it all to be over in order to eat their scavenged meal. Perhaps this is why they came to be disliked. I expect no one enjoyed the feeling of being followed by a bird, lest they might die soon. Yet, let's put things into perspective – it wasn't the ravens killing one another; they simply ate the remains of human battles. They were intelligent enough to work out that groups of men often killed one another. This knowledge meant that ravens have always gone hand in hand with death. In Slavic mythology, it was said that their ultimate home was *Wyraj* (*Vyray*) – the place where birds go in the winter and souls go after death, located in the Tree of Life.

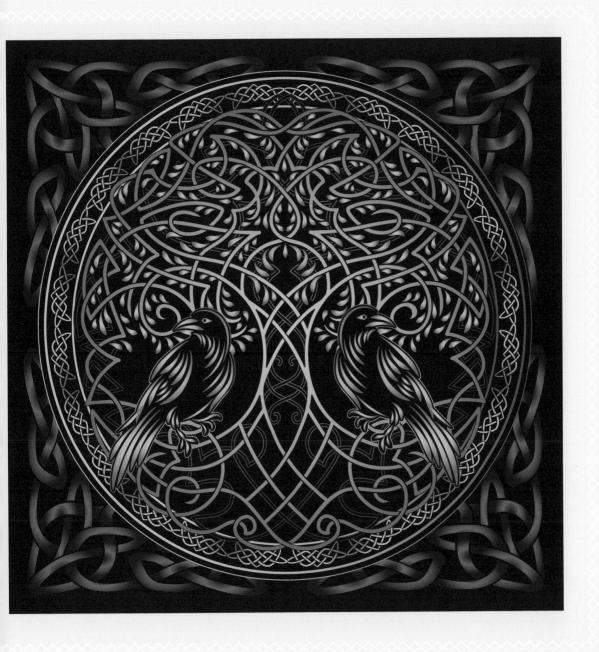

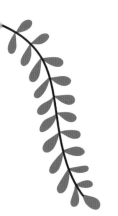

HERBAL TEA MIXES for all kinds of coughs

Getting a cold feels like evidence that my energy is depleted. I am therefore always slightly annoyed with myself for getting ill, as if it could have been prevented – though, really, it is evidence of a change of seasons. Colds and coughs are expected during autumn (and, of course, in the long run, we need them to strengthen our immune system).

These herbal tea blends are variations (often simplifications) of ones I've found in Polish herbal magazines to treat a cough, and which I've found to be effective. In fact, I can personally recommend a three-way remedy for a cold and cough: drinking these herbal teas, as instructed below, along with the three-herb inhalation (opposite) and taking a cough syrup (this could be the onion cough syrup on page 144 , the black radish one on page 69 or one from the pharmacy).

Note:
If you have none of the other ingredients to hand, just an infusion from fresh plantain (Plantago) leaves does wonders to soothe the throat. Plantain can be found on most patches of grass year-round (just make sure it's a clean, natural patch you are picking from with no artificial

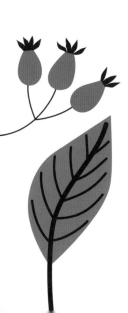

fertilizers used or cars going past). Plantain really is one of the most common, most beneficial and most underused greens of our times.

MIX 1 - ANY COUGH
7 plantain (*Plantago*) leaves – can be greater or ribwort plantain
1 star anise
1 stem of fresh thyme or ½ teaspoon dried thyme
1 teaspoon good-quality honey

MIX 2 - DRY COUGH
7 plantain (*Plantago*) leaves – can be greater or ribwort plantain
1 star anise
1 stem of fresh thyme or ½ teaspoon dried thyme
1 stem of fresh marjoram or ½ teaspoon dried marjoram
1 teaspoon good-quality honey

MIX 3 - WET COUGH
7 plantain (*Plantago*) leaves – can be broadleaf or ribwort plantain
1 star anise
1 stem of fresh thyme or ½ teaspoon dried thyme
3 sage leaves
1 teaspoon good-quality honey

MIX 4 - COUGH WITH RAISED TEMPERATURE
7 plantain (*Plantago*) leaves – can be broadleaf or ribwort plantain
3 rosehips
3 hawthorn berries
1 birch leaf
1 teaspoon good-quality honey

◉ Wash all of the fresh herbs you've foraged gently but thoroughly under running water.

◉ Place in a pan and cover with 400ml/14fl oz/1⅔ cups cold filtered water. Cover the pan and bring to the boil slowly over a low heat. As soon as it starts to boil, turn the heat off.

◉ Leave to infuse for about 10 minutes, so that the drink is still very warm (but not scalding hot) when you pour it into your thermos flask. The drink will continue to infuse slowly in the flask. After 2 hours, strain out the herbs using a sieve and stir in the honey.

◉ Pour it back into your thermos flask to keep warm. Drink throughout the day, until it is finished (three to four times a day).

THREE-HERB INHALATION for the common cold

Many Ukrainian folk songs begin with the hero taking three herbs for one purpose or another. It is not said which herbs they are and the purposes may vary, but the point is that three is a magical number where herbs are concerned. The very first thing I do when I feel a cold coming on is an inhalation. This three-herb inhalation is ideal, but if I don't have all three to hand then I will use whatever I have just to start the cleansing process. You need to do inhalations every day of your cold in order to keep cleansing your respiratory system ...

MAKES 1 INHALATION

1 sprig of fresh thyme
1 sprig of fresh peppermint
1 baby pinecone bud or a small branch
  from pine tree
Towel

◉ Place the three herbs in a large bowl, and place a towel over the bowl.

◉ Pour boiling water over the herbs, holding the towel up on one side.

◉ As soon as you've poured in the water, put your head under the towel and take deep breaths in. Keep your head under the towel for 5–10 minutes.

THE MUCH DREADED YET EXTREMELY EFFECTIVE ONION SYRUP for a sore throat

This is the syrup of my childhood nightmares. I find the taste too sickly sweet to bear. However, it is a medicine and, as such, it's not there to be enjoyed. I could not leave this syrup out of a book on Slavic remedies, because it was the main medicine that I was given as a child at the first sign of a sore throat – we were all given it! Many Poles still swear by the syrup's effectiveness and plenty of people don't even find it horrible any more, as they are so used to it. The lemon juice works to improve the taste and preserve it too.

Note:
This syrup is now recommended for children over three.

MAKES 1 X 250ml/9fl oz BOTTLE

1 large white onion, roughly
   chopped
5–6 tablespoons good-quality
   runny honey
3 tablespoons lemon juice (optional)
250ml/9fl oz sterilized glass jar
250ml/9fl oz sterilized glass bottle

◉ Place the chopped onion in the jar.

◉ Spoon in the honey, making sure the onion is completely covered. Seal the jar with the lid and shake it.

◉ Leave in a warm place for 48 hours, shaking the jar whenever you remember (three times a day would be ideal).

◉ After 48 hours, you will have plenty of syrup. Strain out the onion and pour the syrup into the sterilized bottle. If you would like to add lemon juice, then add it now.

◉ Drink 1 tablespoon three times a day when you feel a sore throat coming on. This syrup is said to lose its potency after 2 weeks. Store in the refrigerator or a cool, dark place.

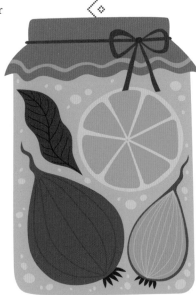

LAYERED FERMENT
for a healthy gut

I came across this *biała ćwikła* ferment in a very old book, where it was just described as a jar full of light-coloured vegetables layered on top of one another and fermented. Fermented foods have an array of health benefits, perhaps the most important one being that they can increase the good bacteria in your gut. You can also drink a shot of the brine when you need it, as a health elixir or hangover cure.

MAKES 1 X 1l/35fl oz JAR

500ml/17fl oz/2 cups warm water from a pre-boiled kettle
1 tablespoon sea salt
1 turnip, peeled and sliced
1 bulb of garlic, cloves separated, peeled and sliced
10–20cm (4–8in) horseradish root, peeled and grated
½ small white cabbage, shredded
2–3 yellow beetroot, peeled and sliced
1l/35fl oz sterilized glass jar

◙ Mix the water with the salt until it has dissolved.

◙ Layer all your sliced vegetables into the jar. Once the jar is full, cover the vegetables in the salty water mixture. Make sure everything is covered; you can place a clean weight on top to keep the vegetables submerged.

◙ Put the jar on a plate, place the lid on loosely and leave at room temperature for 3 days.

◙ After 3 days, make sure everything looks and smells healthy, close the lid securely and keep in the refrigerator. It will keep for about 2 months.

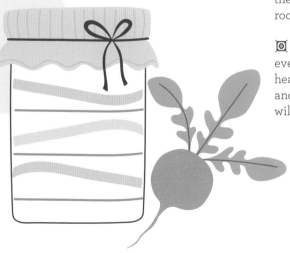

YARROW INFUSION
to settle the stomach

The extremely common and unassuming yarrow (*Achillea millefolium*) is called *krwawnik* in Polish folk stories, which immediately lets us know that it has something to do with the blood – *krew*. In the past, it was used to soothe external wounds and stop bleeding. Taken internally, it was also associated with the blood, as it was used to regulate menstruation. Additionally, it is known to soothe the stomach, which is what I tend to use it for, extremely effectively. Usually, my stomach needs most soothing when I am menstruating. I used to reach for a paracetamol at this time of the month, now I reach for the yarrow.

To dry:
Wash the flower heads under running water and allow to dry naturally in a sieve. Arrange on a baking sheet lined with greaseproof/wax paper and place in the oven at the lowest setting (about 50°C/120°F) for 10–15 minutes. Turn the oven off and allow them to cool down. Keep in a sterilized glass jar for up to 3 months.

SERVES 1

1 tablespoon dried yarrow
250ml/9fl oz/1 cup hot water
  from a pre-boiled kettle
1 teaspoon good-quality honey
  (optional)

◙ Place the yarrow in a teapot or thermos flask and cover with the hot (not boiling) water.

◙ Allow to infuse for about 10 minutes before drinking. Sweeten with honey, if you choose.

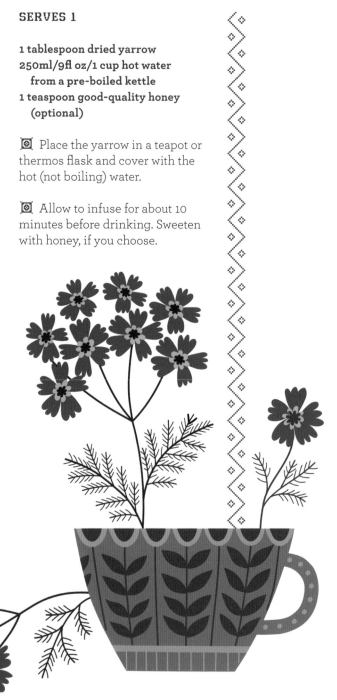

TREE OF LIFE

"A noble tree" still echoes in my ears every time I pass an oak, because it's something that my Babcia Hala always used to say. She was an avid tree lover and hugger.

The axis mundi is where the Earth and the heavens meet and it's how the function of the Slavic Tree of Life – an oak – is often described. Oaks hold a special significance to the Slavs and are a part of our ancient mythology. Lightning likes to strike large oaks, and so it was considered to be the chosen tree of the most powerful Slavic God, Perun – the God of Thunder – who blessed it on a regular basis. Nevertheless, it was Rod, as the forefather of the gods, who was pictured to be living within the cosmic Tree of Life that links all people (which is where Polish words such as *rodzina* – family – and *ród* – race – come from).

According to the mythology, within the Tree of Life there existed another dimension, known as *Wyraj*, a land where it is always spring. The souls rested here between lives. The birds also loved *Wyraj* and stayed here during the winter months, returning in the spring with the souls that were ready to be reborn.

While religions have changed, love for the oak tree has remained. Polish kings were known to hold meetings under certain oak trees. Public courts were also held under the oak's wise branches, to preserve order and help the trial reach its fairest conclusion. Some oaks were so loved and honoured that they were even given names and people would come from far and wide to receive their blessings.

BEET LEAVES
for a headache

Beetroot is the vegetable that's probably most associated with East European cooking, and with good reason. In Poland and the northern East European countries, we eat it year-round in various guises, but we have perhaps forgotten some of its purported healing properties. The juice was used as a cure for sore throats and buzzing in the ears, while the leaves were used to heal headaches. While the small spring beetroot leaves are most suited to making soup, the large autumnal ones are ideal for creating compresses for the head.

MAKES 1 COMPRESS

4 large beetroot leaves
Bowl of warm water from
  a pre-boiled kettle

◉ Remove the stems from the leaves. Wash the leaves under running water, then place in the bowl of warm water.

◉ Lie down. Take the leaves out of the water, allow to drip-dry for a moment, shaking gently, then place them on your forehead, well into your hairline and over your temples and even your eyes.

◉ Close your eyes and relax for 20 minutes.

HOME-FERMENTED APPLE CIDER VINEGAR for all ills

Apples are plentiful in autumn, making this is the ideal time to create something from the surplus that we can use all year long. There are many varieties of cider apples, so you shouldn't have any problems in finding a variety that's locally available. Apple cider vinegar has been made in Poland since ancient times, using the art of fermentation to harness the healing properties of the apples. This ancient Slavic recipe is now hailed as a remedy for everything from blood sugar regulation to bad skin.

Apples have traditionally been used in Slavic folk customs as well as for various health issues. Giving someone an apple was a sign of commitment in certain villages and they even appeared on a wedding branch carried by grooms on their wedding day. In terms of health, apples were often associated with the throat but were also used externally to help with things like cramps and warts. Whatever the regional and historical customs have been, the apple has always been associated with health and beauty.

MAKES 1 X 2l/70fl oz JAR

1l/35fl oz/4¼ cups warm water
    from a pre-boiled kettle
5 tablespoons sugar
1kg/2lb 4oz organic cider apples,
    washed, cored and quartered
2l/70fl oz sterilized glass jar
Gauze
Bottle

◙ Mix the warm water and sugar.

◙ Place the chopped apples in
the jar and cover with the sugar
water. To make sure the apples
are always submerged, you
can place a clean weight on top
(nothing metal).

◙ Cover the jar with a gauze
secured with an elastic band
or piece of string.

◙ Keep the jar at room
temperature, ideally in a
dark corner, for 2–5
weeks, then strain out
the plant matter and pour
the vinegar into a bottle.
Keep it in a cool,
preferably dark place.

APPLE CIDER VINEGAR TONER for a clear complexion

In Poland, apple cider vinegar is
used to create a simple toner for
the skin. Its antibacterial and
anti-fungal properties, as well
as all the probiotics from the
fermentation process, makes it a
wonderful product for removing
impurities, and it's far less
abrasive than alcohol. I use it after
washing my face in the evening.
With distilled water, I would keep
this for up to a month; if you use
normal water from a pre-boiled
kettle, then make a smaller
amount every 3–4 days.

MAKES 1 X 150ml/5fl oz BOTTLE

3 tablespoons apple cider vinegar
100ml/3½fl oz/scant ½ cup distilled
    water from a pre-boiled kettle
8 drops lavender or rose
    essential oil
150ml/5fl oz sterilized glass bottle

◙ Pour all the ingredients into
the sterilized bottle, then shake
vigorously to mix.

◙ Use a cotton pad to wipe your
face in the evening, after cleansing
and before a night balm.

ACORN COFFEE for a caffeine-free energy boost

The fruit of the venerated oak tree (*Quercus*) has had many uses throughout the years. In remote Slavic villages, especially in the south, acorn flour is still mixed with wheat flour to make bread.

Acorns need to be collected after St Michael's day – 29 September – to make sure that they are fully ripe. I would aim to collect them the first week of October and make sure you only collect healthy, whole ones. I've come across various methods of making acorn coffee, some shorter than mine. I like to keep on the safe side and remove as many tannins as possible through leeching, so my method does take some time. But it's worth it for the gorgeous taste and the overall benefits.

Acorn coffee contains magnesium, which we need for hundreds of different bodily functions, including energy release.

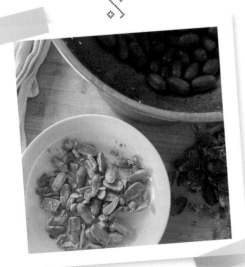

If you are feeling tired, it's possible that your body could be lacking in magnesium. This acorn coffee is a perfect accompaniment to some sunflower seed halva (see page 127).

Note:
Acorns contain vitamin A and too much of this vitamin isn't recommended for pregnant women.

MAKES 1 JAR

500g/1lb 2oz acorns
Plenty of filtered or mineral water
Sterilized glass jar

◉ Collect the acorns, take off their hats if they still have them on and place in a large bowl filled with 1l/35fl oz/4¼ cups of filtered or mineral water. Cover and leave for 24 hours. Change the water halfway through.

◉ Take the acorns out of the water and place in a saucepan. Cover with fresh, filtered or mineral water and bring to the boil. Turn the heat down and simmer for 10 minutes, then turn the heat off and allow to cool for at least 2 hours.

◉ Take the acorns out of the water and place on paper towels to dry.

◙ Use the flat blade of a knife to lightly crush the acorns and remove their outer shells. Halve the acorns, cut off any black bits and scrape off as much of their skins as you can.

◙ Now, to remove some more of their tannins, place the shelled acorns in a bowl and cover with boiling water. Cover and leave to stand for 5–10 minutes. Drain and repeat a few times until the water is almost clear (I usually repeat about five times). Dry with paper towels.

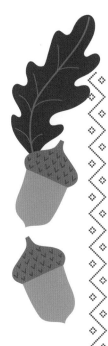

◙ Using a large knife, chop the acorns as small as you can and place in a dry frying pan. Toast gently, stirring regularly, for about 8–10 minutes. Allow to cool and transfer to a jar. The coffee will keep for about 3 months.

◙ Before making your acorn coffee your favourite way, grind the acorn bits in a coffee grinder or a powerful blender.

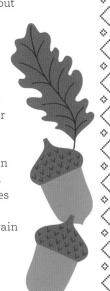

◙ Boil 2–3 tablespoons of acorn coffee with 300ml/10½ fl oz/1¼ cups filtered water for 10 minutes in a small pan, then cover and allow to stand for 5 minutes. Strain out the acorns, add milk and a teaspoon of honey or sugar if you like.

ACORN AND HONEY BISCUITS for a good mood

Over the centuries, acorn flour was used in bread in times of famine. It may therefore have had negative associations and been unnecessarily overlooked at other times in history. This is a shame, as acorns have a unique, rich flavour that's not found anywhere else. Once you have shelled the acorns, they should be smooth and caramel in colour, hinting at that flavour you'll find when you cook with them.

Magnesium is one of the benefits of acorns. Sometimes magnesium is even used to help treat depression. Of course, I do not recommend acorn biscuits instead of any medication if you have been diagnosed with depression, but it is fair to say that they can lift the mood.

Recipes for acorn biscuits have been found in old, Polish cookbooks, with honey often used as a sweetener. This is my own version of those recipes.

Note:
Acorns contain vitamin A and too much of this vitamin isn't recommended for pregnant women.

MAKES 12-14 COOKIES

120g/4¼oz (peeled weight) acorns, peeled (see pages 150–1) and very finely chopped
100g/3½oz salted butter
8 tablespoons good-quality honey
120g/4¼oz/1 cup plain/all-purpose flour
½ teaspoon bicarbonate of soda/baking soda
½ teaspoon baking powder
50g/1¾oz/½ cup barley flakes or rolled oats, ground (or oatmeal)
1 small egg, lightly beaten
1 teaspoon vanilla extract
1 teaspoon vodka (can be flavoured)
1 tablespoon sesame seeds

◉ Treat the acorns as when making acorn coffee (see page 150), but do not toast them. Do grind them up as small as possible – they should be the consistency of breadcrumbs.

◉ Preheat the oven to 200°C/400°F/Gas mark 6 and line a baking sheet with greaseproof/wax paper.

◉ Melt the butter with the honey in a small saucepan over a medium heat. Once it's melted, add the ground acorns. Cook over a low heat for about 5 minutes, stirring regularly with a wooden spoon.

◉ Transfer the mixture to a large bowl. Sift in the flour, the bicarbonate of soda and baking powder, then add the ground barley or oats and mix with your hand. Add the egg, vanilla extract and vodka. Mix again with your hands to combine thoroughly and form a dough ball.

◉ Take chunks the size of walnuts from the ball and roll them with wet hands.

◉ Place each one on the lined baking sheet and flatten slightly into a circle. Press some sesame seeds into the top of each cookie. Use the bottom of the cookies to mop up any spilled sesame seeds.

◉ Bake for approximately 15 minutes, or until golden brown. Allow to cool on the baking sheet for 10 minutes before transferring to a wire rack to cool completely.

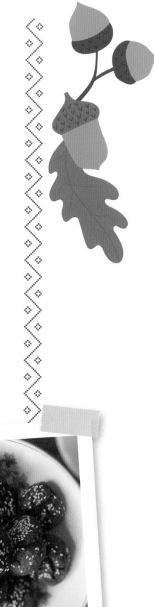

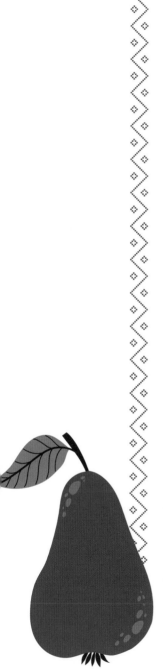

SPICED MILLET *BABKA* WITH STEWED PEARS for a healthy glow and getting rid of vampires

I like to think of a *babka* as the Slavic celebration of the female form – the more rounded the better! *Babkas* are known all over Eastern Europe mostly as cakes, though they can also be savoury, made from potato. This breakfast *babka* has become one of my favourites. I love millet in this recipe, as there is still some bite to it, even when it's been soaked overnight. Millet is one of the oldest *kasza* grains cultivated on these lands and its nutty flavour is a perfect match for earthy spices, while the raisins give this babka a delightful sweetness. Millet is high in the vitamin niacin, which is vital for the skin and organ function.

MAKES 4 INDIVIDUAL BABKAS

FOR THE BABKAS
400ml/14fl oz/1¾ cups milk
250g/9oz/1⅓ cups millet, rinsed
100g/3½oz/1 cup raisins
2 tablespoons honey
½ teaspoon ground cinnamon
½ teaspoon ground cardamom
Pinch of salt and black pepper

FOR THE STEWED FRUIT
4 pears, peeled and sliced
¼ teaspoon ground cinnamon
¼ teaspoon ground cardamom
1 tablespoon water
1 tablespoon honey

FOR THE TOPPING:
Hazelnuts, toasted and broken up
    into smaller pieces

◉ The night before, pour the milk into a saucepan, add the millet and bring to the boil, then turn the heat down and simmer for 20 minutes.

◉ Add all the other babka ingredients, cover and leave for 10 minutes.

◉ Rinse four cereal bowls in cold water and place in the refrigerator for 10 minutes.

◉ Divide the still warm kasza between the bowls and leave to cool completely before placing in the refrigerator.

◉ In the morning, make the stewed fruit: place the pears in a saucepan, sprinkle with the spices, add the tablespoon of water and stew for about 5 minutes. Add the honey at the end.

◉ Carefully turn your bowls over onto serving plates to remove the *babkas* and serve with the stewed fruit on the side and the toasted hazelnuts sprinkled on top.

THE VAMPIRE AND SAINT MICHAEL – (A Cossack story)

In a faraway land, there lived two neighbours: one rich, one poor. A time came when the poor man had nothing to eat, so he went to his rich neighbour's house, greeted him politely and asked him kindly for one silver rouble.

"Who will stand as surety for thee?" asked the rich man.

"I know not of any man, yet, perchance, God and St Michael will be my sureties", and he pointed at the icon in the corner. Then, the icon of St Michael spoke to the rich man and said, "Lend it to him and God will repay thee!"

"I'll lend it", said the rich man. The poor man thanked him and returned to his home happy. Yet the rich man was not content that God should give him back his loan in blessings. He grew resentful. Finally, he went over to the poor man's house and shouted: "Thou son of a dog, why hast thou not brought me back my money?!"

The poor man's wife burst into tears and told him that he had died some time ago, yet the rich man was still angry. He took the icon of St Michael and started beating it. He was stamping on the statue when a young man stopped him and said: "Beat him not, and I will give you a silver rouble", and he ran home and begged to borrow one from his father.

The young man washed the statue and placed it in the middle of some flowers. His three uncles were rich sea merchants. When they were preparing for their next voyage, the young man asked them to let him come on board to sell boards and laths. They laughed but allowed him on board. He took the icon of St Michael and they departed.

They sailed a short distance and they sailed a long distance, til at last they came to another tsardom, a place shrouded in grief, for the Tsar's daughter had been possessed by an evil spirit and lay dead in a coffin. In his despair, the Tsar ordered someone into the church every night to read from the holy book over her, promising half his tsardom to the person who exorcised the demon. Yet every morning, only bones were left. He lost so many of his subjects that the Tsar ordered all foreign merchants to go into the church. All ended up as bones.

Then came the turn of the uncles. The first one cried and asked his young nephew to go instead. The nephew refused, until Saint Michael spoke to him: "Go and fear not! Stand in the middle of the church, fenced with thy laths and boards, and take with thee a basket full of pears. When she rushes at thee, scatter the pears, and it will take her till cockcrow to pick them all up. But do thou go on reading thy prayers all the time, and do not look up."

He did as he was told. In the dead of night, the Tsarina arose from her coffin and came toward him hissing. She leaped upon the boards and made to grab at him and fell back. He scattered the pears. All through the church they rolled and she went after them. At the first cockcrow, she went back into her coffin. And when the people came to sweep away his bones, he was still there, reading his prayers.

The second uncle's turn came and he too cried and pleaded with his nephew. The young man refused until Saint Michael spoke to him again. This time he was instructed to take a basket of nuts with him. Once again, the undead Tsarina jumped onto the boards to get him, then went dutifully after the nuts and tried to pick them all up until the first cockcrow. He was alive in the morning.

The third uncle's turn came and again St Michael told the youth to go, but this time the instructions he

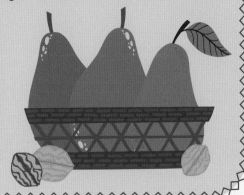

gave were different: "Fence thyself about with thy boards, sprinkle thyself all about with holy water, incense thyself with holy incense, and take me with thee. And the moment she leaves her coffin, jump quickly into it. And whatever she may say to thee, and however she may implore thee, let her not get into it again until she says to thee, 'My consort!'"

So that night, he stood in the middle of the church, fenced himself about with his boards, strewed consecrated poppy seeds around him, incensed himself with holy incense and read. A tempest arose outside. Then he heard hissing from the coffin, so the youth quickly hid himself so that he could jump into the coffin while the Tsarina rushed the boards once more.

She darted madly from one corner of the church to the other, seeking him everywhere. Eventually she looked in the coffin and, seeing him in there with the statue of Saint Michael beside him, she screeched: "Come down, come down! I'll try and catch thee no more!" But he only prayed to God, and never uttered a word. Then the cock crowed once, "Come down, come down, my consort!" cried the Tsarina. Then he came down, and they both fell on their knees and wept and prayed to God, giving thanks, because He had mercy on them both.

At dawn, crowds of people, with the Tsar at the head of them, came to the church.

Then the Tsar rejoiced and gave the young man half his kingdom, but the merchants departed in their ships, with their nephew on board.

The Tsar's daughter grew sadder by the day. The Tsar was starting to despair, when one night he had a dream and a voice told him the reason for his daughter's sadness. The next day, the Tsar asked her, "Do you love the man who saved you?" and Tsarina replied "Yes". And so they sent for the kind-hearted, brave youth, who married the Tsarina and they lived a wonderful life together.

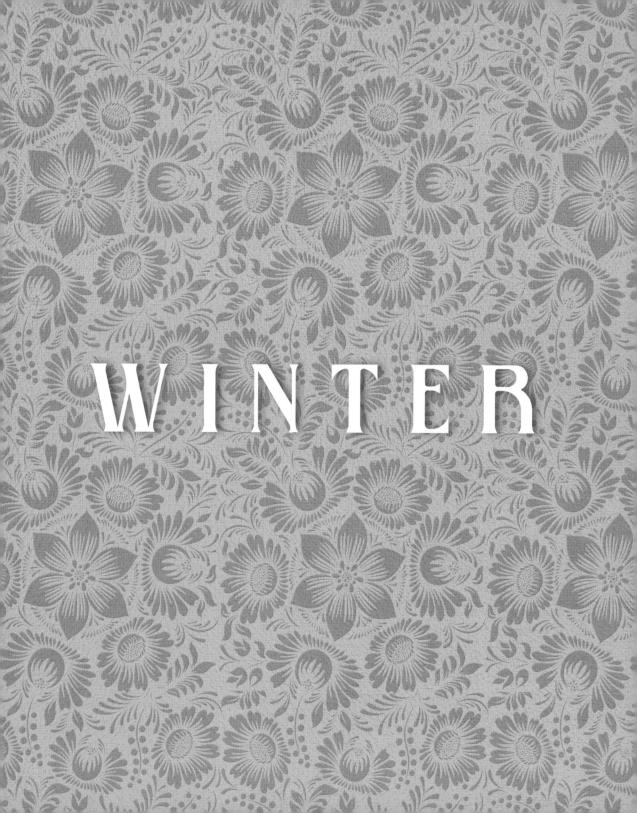

WINTER

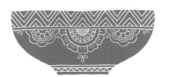

Sparkling fresh snow is one of those magical things that has the power to turn a monotonous sea of Communist blocks into a gleaming wonderland. Winters used to be so full of snow when I was child that we would make igloos in the playground. During those happy moments, we ice skated and went sledding and even skiing on a nearby (very small) hill. Life became exciting.

Then, all of sudden, the north wind would bring a chill from Siberia, temperatures dropped to below minus 40 and we couldn't leave the house for days on end. We'd pray for a bit of warmth, but too much warmth and then it all turned to slush. Our shiny new world melted, leaving exhaust-blackened slush piles on the sides of the road. The many faces of winter.

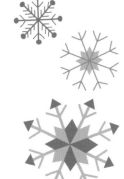

Living close to the earth and its rhythms sounds idyllic, yet we must remember that the reality has always been quite harsh for the Slavic lands. That harshness, those challenges, are a part of life, and we all must face them in one form or another – Baba Yaga the crone (see page 190) is here to remind us of that. In the olden days, winter was a time of rest for the people who worked on the land. Yes, it's fun to frolic in the snow, but we're also left with many long evenings to look closely at ourselves. Some of us aren't ready,

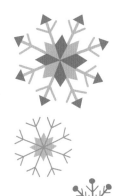

of course, and will spend our time drinking away the shadows. But the invitation to be courageous always remains … Once we are ready, we can light and warm our own paths with some simple Slavic winter rituals.

One way to spend long, bitterly cold evenings is to sit around a large kitchen table with a few simple tools and make things with our hands. Slavic folk arts use things such as paper and rye straw to make decorations for the home, and I find them to be an effective way of relaxing the mind. Once we get into the rhythm with our hands, we get into an almost meditative state and our minds are free to calmly contemplate.

Among the peasants, many pagan winter traditions have survived, intermingling with the Christian beliefs at Christmas-time. In Poland, Czechia and Slovakia, Christmas Eve is considered magical. In the past, it was commonly believed that on Christmas Eve our dead ancestors were among us, that animals could speak in human voices and that lakes and rivers flowed with wine. At dawn, pine trees were sought from the forests, and used to decorate the home, often being hung from the ceiling.

Once the magic of Christmas-time is over, keeping the spirits high can be a challenge. In Poland at this time of year, the nobility would organize a *kulig*, a horse-drawn sleighride party, where they would party hop around the nearby

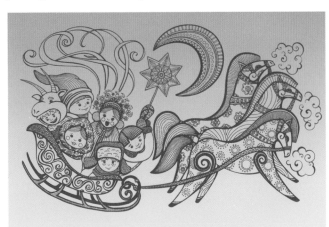

nobles' houses, eating and drinking lavishly everywhere they went. Folkloric (peasant) traditions were far humbler and more centered on the home. These are what I will focus on in this chapter, for they are what I believe will bring us closer to the earth's rhythms and to ourselves. I have searched out Slavic winter foods, traditions, stories and rituals from all over the eastern lands and times past, in the hope that they will bring us health, strength and inner peace when we need them most.

In terms of food, it's easy to overindulge during all the time spent at home, especially because this is the time of year when we want comfort foods. I believe that this is a key time to focus on maintaining a healthy gut, so that it can thrive and cope with the extra load and heavier foods. This chapter starts with a few suggestions of how we can do just that.

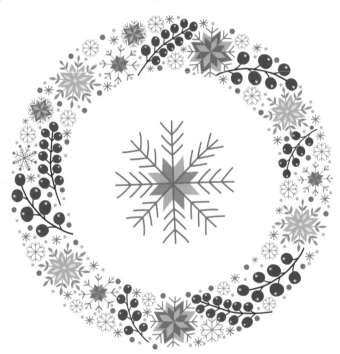

OVERNIGHT FLAXSEED to aid digestion

This is an old remedy that my grandad used to swear by, as he often suffered with stomach complaints. The water my Babcia Ziuta used was warm, but science now dictates that the water should be tepid or cold, which thankfully makes the mixture a whole lot less gloopy. As my mother always explains, flaxseeds need to be freshly ground for us to obtain their full benefits. She has a little hand mill especially for this purpose. You could use a coffee or spice grinder as well, of course, or even a pestle and mortar. While people who take this flaxseed mixture religiously do it year-round, I think it's perfectly suited to the excesses of the Christmas period.

SERVES 1

1 tablespoon flaxseeds,
   freshly ground
150ml/5fl oz/²/₃ cup tepid water
   from a pre-boiled kettle

TO SERVE
3 tablespoons thick live yogurt
1 tablespoon good-quality runny
   honey
1 tablespoon dried fruit, such
   as raisins or finely diced prunes
   or apricots

◙ Place the flaxseeds in your mill, grinder or pestle and mortar and grind to a powder.

◙ Transfer the flaxseed powder to a small bowl or cup and pour the tepid water over. Mix to combine. Cover with a small plate and leave overnight to soak.

◙ In the morning, drink what's left of the liquid first thing, then mix the rest of the mixture with yogurt and honey and eat with dried fruit on top.

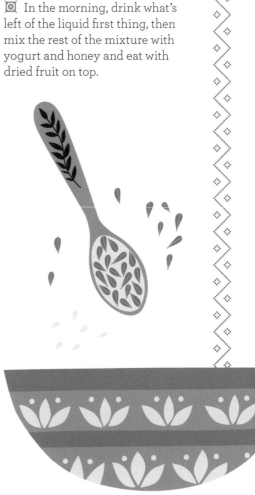

OAT AND BARLEY PANCAKES WITH CINNAMON BUTTER
for a healthy gut

Across the Eastern lands, pancakes are much loved and eaten in various guises. In ancient times, pancakes were used in pagan rites as a symbol of plentifulness and protection – the round shape was a symbol of the sun. In deepest Belarus, a shepherd was given a pancake when he took his herd out in the spring, and in some villages, fortunes are still told by reading pancake shapes (there's no need to make them all uniform if you want to be a fortune teller).

Both oats and barley are now proven to create an environment in the gut where beneficial bacteria can thrive. From experience, I can say that they also give you a full, happy and warm feeling from the inside, which lasts for the entire morning.

SERVES 4-6

200g/7oz/2 cups rolled oats
200g/7oz/2 cups barley flakes
4 tablespoons caster/granulated
    sugar
¼ teaspoon salt
2 tablespoons plain/all-purpose
    flour
3 eggs
220ml/8fl oz/scant 1 cup milk
100g/3½oz butter (salted
    or unsalted), softened
Mild oil, for frying
1 teaspoon ground cinnamon
2 tablespoons runny honey

◙ Place the oats and the barley in a food processor and grind into a rough flour. Add the sugar and salt, then blitz a few more times.

◙ Add the flour, eggs, milk and half of the butter and blend thoroughly. Allow the batter to rest for 10–15 minutes.

◙ Pour a thin film of oil into a frying pan over a medium heat. Once the oil is hot (you can test it by adding a tiny bit of batter to the pan; if it starts bubbling almost immediately, then it's ready), spoon the mixture into the pan in batches – 1 tablespoon per pancake – and fry the pancakes for 2–3 minutes on each side. Remove onto a paper towel.

◙ Melt the remainder of the butter in a small pan. Add the cinnamon and honey and allow to heat through, then take off the heat. Once the pancakes are ready, serve them with the cinnamon butter.

SPROUTING RYE PORRIDGE WITH CRANBERRIES for inner and outer radiance

Porridge is one of the oldest cooked foods known to man. Eating it on a crisp winter morning makes you feel ready to face the frosty day ahead. The warmth within is reflected on the outside, as this porridge will give you a radiant complexion thanks to the combination of vitamins and minerals found in both the rye and the sour dried cranberries.

This wonderful winter breakfast is inspired by the Russian-style baked porridge in Darra Goldstein's *Beyond the North Wind*. This has become a winter favourite and I have put my own spin on it. While nut and grain milks may seem a modern invention, I found a recipe for almond milk in a very old Polish cookbook from the 19th century, so it's clearly a returning trend.

Note:
It's easy for the rye berries to develop mould, so we need to be vigilant about changing the water and the paper towels that they will be sprouting on.

SERVES 2

FOR THE SPROUTING BERRIES
200g/7oz rye berries

FOR THE PORRIDGE
200g/7oz sprouting rye berries
2 tablespoons dried cranberries
200ml/7fl oz/scant 1 cup warm
    almond or oat milk
3 tablespoons honey
½ teaspoon salt

TO SERVE
1 tablespoon butter (salted or
    unsalted) or butter alternative
2 tablespoons double/heavy cream
2 teaspoons good-quality runny
    honey

◙ Place the rye berries in a bowl and cover with water. Cover the bowl with a plate and leave for 48 hours, changing the water every 12 hours.

◙ Strain the rye berries and place them on a baking sheet lined with a double layer of paper towels. Spray the paper towels with water, and leave them in a warm place. The berries should start to sprout in 2–3 days. Change the paper towels every day.

◙ Preheat the oven to 180°C/350°F/ Gas mark 4.

◙ Place all the ingredients for the porridge in an ovenproof dish and mix well with a wooden spoon. Cover and place in the oven for 45 minutes.

◙ Remove from the oven and stir in a tablespoon of butter, then serve with a dollop of cream and a drizzle of honey.

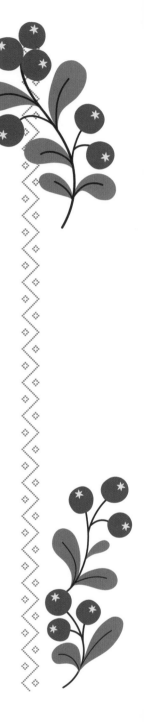

THE MYTH OF MARZANNA

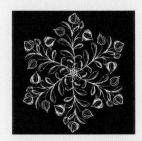

In Slavic folklore, Marzanna was the Goddess of Winter, also known as Morena, Mara and Mora, and even Śmierć, which literally means "death" in Polish. Throughout the ages, Marzanna's role has diminished somewhat because, to the earliest Slavs, she had many functions, not only those of winter, but also to do with life and fertility. The Polish name Marzanna, in fact, comes from *Marzec* – the month of March. Some folk songs call her the Goddess of Life and Death, while others show her association with the rivers and tell her to swim to her lover, Jasiek (diminutive of the god Jaryło). Despite our current one-dimensional interpretation of Marzanna as the Goddess of Winter, she was one of the most venerated and widely worshipped gods in ancient times. Most often seen as a woman in white, Marzanna's traditional attire is, in fact, a wedding gown. She was also known to carry a key to the seasons.

Legend has it that Marzanna was born to Perun, God of Thunder, and Mokosh, Goddess of Life (who, true to her nature, mothered many of the old Slavic gods and goddesses). Some stories claim that her twin brother was Jaryło (also Jarowit or Jarun), whom she was separated from at birth. Later on, Marzanna and Jaryło fell in love and she gave him her key to the seasons. However, Jaryło was unfaithful, so Marzanna changed her mind about the key and sought revenge on her lover. Some say she poisoned Jaryło and as punishment, she was banished from the lands of the gods. In this version of the story, Marzanna and Jaryło could no longer exist at the same time. Marzanna therefore ruled winter and Jaryło was forever born again in the spring.

The ritual drowning of Marzanna as a call for the end of winter – which happens on the spring equinox – takes place in many Slavic villages. Even though the Church distinctly forbade this pagan ritual, many villagers ignored the edict and stubbornly continued to drown the doll, a tradition which continues to this very day (see page 36).

SLAVIC POPPY SEED ROLLS for serenity

Often seen with poppy flowers in her hair, Mokosh was the ancient Slavic patron Goddess of Women and Children, also associated with poppy seeds. She embodies the love we Slavs have for this tiny full-stop of a seed, which in Polish is called *mak*. Indeed, you can find it in various cakes, buns and even pasta dishes – but be warned, when we use poppy seeds, we don't just sprinkle them meagrely over bread products; we tend to use them in large quantities. Poppy seeds are used the most lavishly at Christmas, and often quite a few of the thirteen dishes on the Christmas table include them. I find poppy seed cakes – *makowiec* – to have an ever so slightly relaxing effect, but only when we eat them in large amounts, like we tend to during this time of the year.

Note:
While we never had any warnings growing up, I believe that children should not consume this cake in huge amounts, as poppies can have traces of opiates in them (Spanish ones are reputed to have the most).

SERVES 20

30g/1oz fresh yeast
120ml/4fl oz/½ cup warm milk
4 tablespoons caster/granulated sugar
500g/1lb 2oz/3¾ cups plain/all-purpose flour
100g/3½oz butter (salted or unsalted), melted
2 egg yolks
1 teaspoon vanilla sugar
1 tablespoon rapeseed/canola oil
Pinch of salt
1 teaspoon spirytus or vodka
200g/7oz icing/1½ cups confectioners' sugar
Juice of 1 lemon

FOR THE FILLING
400g/14oz/2¾ cups poppy seeds
100g/3½oz/1 cup almond flakes, gently toasted
50g/1¾oz walnuts, crushed
2–3 drops almond extract
2 eggs
50g/1¾oz/½ cup raisins soaked in 50ml/2fl oz rum
10 tablespoons good-quality runny honey

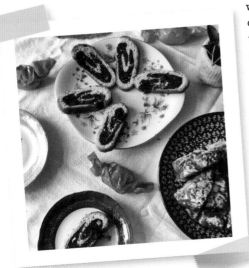

◙ To make the filling, first prep the poppy seeds. Place them in a saucepan, cover in boiling water from a kettle – about 1cm (½in) above the seeds – and bring to the boil. Reduce the heat and simmer for about 30 minutes. Leave to stand overnight.

◙ In the morning, drain the poppyseeds through a sieve, then blitz them in a food processor until they start releasing their milk. This could take up to 30 minutes – you'll see they get lighter and eventually turn into one mass.

◙ Preheat the oven to 190°C/375°F/Gas mark 5 and line a baking sheet with greaseproof/wax paper.

◙ Add all the other ingredients for the filling to the food processor. Depending on the texture you want, you can blend everything together for another couple of minutes, or just mix the other ingredients in with a spoon if you want a chunkier texture.

◙ For the dough, in a large bowl, crumble the yeast into the warm milk, mix with 1 teaspoon of the sugar and leave in a warm place for 10 minutes to activate the yeast.

◙ Add all the other dough ingredients and mix together with your hand. Knead for a few minutes.

◙ Cover your bowl with a dish towel and leave in a warm place to rise for 1–1½ hours.

◙ Place on a floured surface and knead for a moment, incorporating any flour you need into the dough. Roll into a rectangle, about 25 x 15cm (10 x 6in) and 1cm (½in) thick.

◙ Spread your poppy-seed filling in the middle, leaving a 2.5cm (1in) gap all the way around it.

◙ Roll your *makowiec* tightly, starting from one of the long sides and tucking the corners into the short sides as you go.

◙ Place it on the lined baking sheet and wrap it twice in the paper, leaving a gap the size of your finger (for the roll to grow).

◙ Bake for about 40 minutes. Leave to cool then serve sliced.

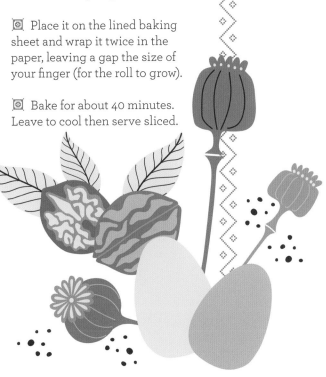

ANCIENT SLAVIC FLATBREAD WITH THREE SEEDS for all-round health and beauty

The ancient Slavs used to make *podpłomyki* – flatbreads – on hot stones in the fire. I imagine they tasted delicious prepared in this way and presumably slightly charred as a result. Nowadays, I find the quickest way to make them is in a frying pan on the stove. The simplest recipe involves just flour, salt and water, although I like to add a mix of three seeds that both enhances the flavour profile and the health benefits of the *podpłomyki*. I don't think it's too far-fetched to believe that other Slavic cooks would have done this before me. I would recommend you make more of this seed mix to use as a topping for other dishes too, such as salads and soups.

All seeds are packed with healthy vitamins and minerals that our bodies need so badly in the wintertime. Caraway is known to be antibacterial and to promote a healthy digestive tract, sunflower seeds keep your heart healthy and sesame seeds promote beautiful skin and hair.

MAKES 6-8 FLATBREADS

1 teaspoon caraway seeds
1 teaspoon sesame seeds
1 teaspoon sunflower seeds
250g/9oz/1¾ cups wholemeal/
   whole-wheat flour
¼ teaspoon salt
120–130ml/4fl oz/½ cup hot water
   from a pre-boiled kettle

◙ Toast the seeds in a dry frying pan, stirring often, until they start to release a nutty smell. Transfer to a pestle and mortar and roughly crush.

◙ Put the crushed seeds, flour and salt in a large bowl and mix to combine. Start adding the water with one hand while mixing with the other. Once it's all come together, stop adding the water (you may not need all of it).

◙ Knead the dough for a few minutes, then divide it into six to eight even portions, rolling them into balls as you go.

◙ Roll out each ball on a lightly floured surface, then fry in a dry frying pan over a medium-high heat for about 2 minutes each side, then the first side again for a further 30 seconds to finish.

GARLIC ON RYE
for a serious immunity boost

If ever anyone is starting to sneeze or feel croaky or tired, they should be immediately offered a piece of rye bread, liberally buttered, with a crushed garlic clove on top, and then sent to bed. In my youth, the remedy also included a drink of warm milk, with a teaspoon of honey and half a teaspoon of butter that formed a delicious golden puddle inside the mug. I have always loved this comforting remedy for a cold. However, I have sadly developed a milk allergy, and modern science has found that milk increases phlegm, so only the garlic on rye remains of my childhood cure. Now and again, I feel a craving for this, and I immediately listen to my body, as I know it's telling me that my immune system needs a boost.

You may want to follow this remedy with a little bit of parsley in order to neutralize the garlic smell, which may otherwise haunt you for a couple of days.

SERVES 1

1 garlic clove
Pinch of sea salt
1 slice of dark rye sourdough
1 teaspoon butter (salted or unsalted)
A little chopped fresh parsley (optional)

◙ Crush the garlic clove with the flat side of a knife, then sprinkle it with salt. Use the sharp edge to cut it, then the flat edge to crush it again. Repeat a few times, until you have a garlic paste of sorts.

◙ Spread the rye bread with the butter, followed by the garlic paste and a sprinkle of parsley, if using. Eat and hop into bed.

SLOW-COOKED BEETROOT BARSZCZ STEW WITH HORSERADISH for vitality

An old Polish lady (who studied chemistry at Oxford with Margaret Thatcher and became an avid beekeeper in her later years) once told me that the food often shows us what it's good for. The example she gave me was walnuts, which, she pointed out, look like a brain and are beneficial to the brain. Following on from this theory, it's interesting to note that blood-red beetroot improves blood flow and blood pressure. It is also known to help fight heart disease, and, if you've ever held a cooked, juicy beetroot in your hand, you will not be able to deny the similarity between the root vegetable and our vital organ: the heart.

In folk wisdom, beetroot has been known to give us strength and vitality. Beetroot and sage rinses were used to heal sore throats, while beetroot leaves were used to heal a headache (see page 148). Moreover, beetroot was also used to attract love through magical rituals.

Horseradish was used in folk medicine long before it was used to flavour food. It is known to soothe pain, help digestion and act as an antibiotic to fight infection. Babcia Ziuta would use the leaves as a compress to soothe rheumatic pain.

Together, beetroot and horseradish are a typically Slavic flavour combination. Here, they meet in a warming and delicious *barszcz* winter stew.

Note:
I like to use lardons in this recipe, as an age-old peasant method of creating depth of flavour, but for a vegetarian version, you can skip them and swap the chicken stock for vegetable stock. I also use a slow cooker for this barszcz *stew, as it's extremely energy efficient. However, you can also use a large pan over a low heat and cook for 2 hours rather than the 4 I indicate in this recipe.*

SERVES 4

2 large or 4 medium beetroots, peeled and diced
1 bay leaf
1 teaspoon allspice berries
½ teaspoon peppercorns
1.5l/52fl oz/6½ cups water
50g/1¾oz bacon lardons
3 tablespoons cold-pressed rapeseed/canola oil
1 tablespoon peeled and grated horseradish root (or 2 tablespoons horseradish sauce)
1 leek, finely chopped
40g/1½oz celeriac/celery root or 1 celery stalk, finely chopped

2–3 carrots, peeled and grated

100g/3½oz beetroot stalks and
  leaves if fresh-looking
  (otherwise cabbage or other
  greens, shredded)

400g/14oz can of chopped tomatoes

2–3 tomatoes, chopped, or another
  400g/14oz can of chopped
  tomatoes

2 large potatoes, peeled and diced

250ml/9fl oz/1 cup chicken or
  vegetable stock

400g/14oz can of butter beans or
  cannellini beans, drained

Juice of 1 lemon

1 teaspoon salt

1 tablespoon sugar

Black and white pepper

TO SERVE

2 tablespoons finely chopped fresh
  dill or parsley

4 tablespoons sour cream
  (optional)

Bread

◙ Place the diced beetroot in the slow cooker with the bay leaf, allspice berries and peppercorns. Cover with the water.

◙ In a frying pan, fry the lardons in a bit of rapeseed oil until slightly crispy. Add to the slow cooker.

◙ Add more rapeseed oil to the pan and fry the horseradish root (if using), stirring for 5 minutes, then add to the slow cooker.

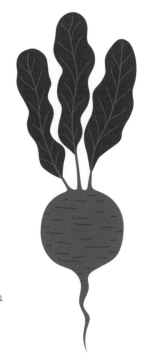

◙ Add more rapeseed oil to the frying pan and fry the leek, celeriac and carrots for about 10 minutes, or until softened, stirring regularly, then add to the slow cooker.

◙ Add the beetroot stalks and leaves, canned tomatoes, fresh tomatoes, potatoes and stock. Place the lid on and cook for 2–2½ hours on low.

◙ Add the beans, lemon juice, salt and sugar, and season with black and white pepper. At this point, add the creamed horseradish sauce, if you didn't use fresh horseradish. Cook for another 2–2½ hours on low.

◙ At the end, taste and adjust the seasoning, then serve with dill or parsley on top and sour cream on the side, if you like. Any good bread works brilliantly with this.

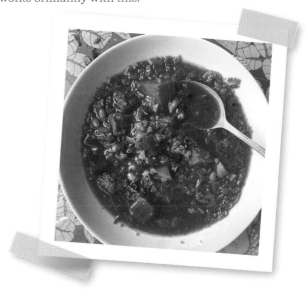

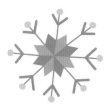

ANIMAL-SHAPED VOTIVE BREADS for New Year celebrations

Christmas and New Year celebrations were considered special to the Slavs, as they were taken to symbolize the new year to come. There is an old Polish saying that goes *Jaki nowy rok, taki cały rok*, which translates as "the whole year, like the New Year". During the Polish Christmas feast, you are encouraged to try all 13 dishes on the table. In fact, folk wisdom tells us that if you don't try one, something will be missing in the year to come. In the new year, you were expected to rise early, to avoid laziness in the year to come, and wash yourself in a basin of cold water, where you'd find a coin – for abundance, naturally.

Votive bread was also used symbolically. Huge plaited breads were made for Christenings by the godmother to the child (or she would pay someone to make one instead, if she wasn't confident in her baking skills), which were meant to show how big and strong the baby would grow. In some areas, you would bake goose breads to give to wedding guests at the reception.

New Year Slavic rituals also varied from one region to the next. In some areas, girls would bake *ferfenuchy* – small, spicy carrot cakes the shape and size of walnuts – which were given to any visiting bachelors. These cakes could also be used for fortune telling – you would throw them up in the air and the girls would catch as many as they could (presumably using a skirt or apron). If the amount they caught was even, that girl would get married in the coming year; if it was odd, she would remain a bachelorette. The animal shapes, on the other hand, were baked to bring health and vitality to the animals in the small holding. Until relatively recently, before land was swapped for apartments in Communist blocks, most households would own a few useful animals, such as hens, goats, pigs or cattle. The animals baked were therefore individual to that household's needs in the coming year. You can use this fun activity to represent the pets you already own or would like to own in the coming year too. Traditionally, they were given to children to eat.

MAKES 2-4

120g/4¼oz/1 cup strong bread flour, plus more for dusting
120g/4¼oz/1 cup light rye flour
Large pinch of salt
7g/¼oz fast-action/instant active dried yeast

60g/2¼oz/3⅔ cups golden
   caster/granulated sugar
1 egg
100ml/3½fl oz/scant ½ cup
   whole milk
½ teaspoon vanilla extract
30g/1oz unsalted butter, melted

◙ In a large bowl, mix together the two flours, salt, yeast and sugar.

◙ In another bowl, lightly beat the egg, then add the milk, butter and vanilla extract. Whisk gently, then start adding to the flour mixture with one hand while bringing the dough together with the other. The dough is too wet to call this kneading, so rather, beat it with your hand, so that it all comes together into one mass. After a few minutes, cover with a clean dish towel and leave in a warm place to rise for 2 hours. After the 2 hours, it should have risen, but it won't have doubled in size as it would if you had been using just wheat flour.

◙ Preheat the oven to 180°C/350°F/Gas mark 4.

◙ Place the dough on a heavily floured surface and knead vigorously, incorporating as much flour as you need to in order for the dough to be workable.

◙ After about 5–6 minutes of kneading, split the dough into however many portions you need.

Each person gets one portion to create their own animal. You can then split the dough further to make heads and tails. Make sure that whatever strong features the animal has are accentuated. You can place the dough over a wooden spoon or rolling pin and the like to create two sets of legs, so that the creature can stand up (bake with the wooden utensil). Keep it simple, as they will change shape and expand as they bake.

◙ Bake for 30–35 minutes until golden.

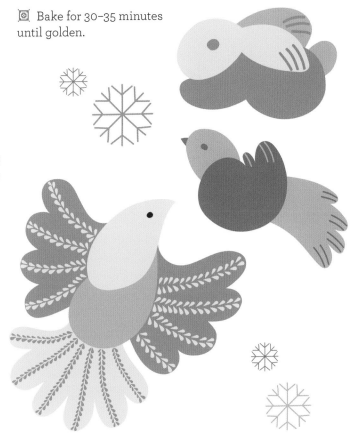

WOLVES IN SLAVIC FOLKLORE

While wolves have gained a reputation for being bloody and ravenous in more recent tales, in old Slavic folklore the wolf was seen as a force for good and a creature to be revered. Some Slavic pagan gods and goddesses are associated with wolves. Dadźbóg (Dazhbog), the Sun God who was born every morning and died every night as the sun set, was one of the few gods worshipped unanimously throughout the Slavic lands and appeared in the form of the white wolf. Veles, the God of the Underworld, who takes care of the animals of the forest, was also known to shapeshift into a wolf.

Werewolves, on the other hand, were said to be creatures who were either born half man or turned by a witch's curse. There are many folk stories of family members who were discovered to be a werewolf. I have also heard a tale of a werewolf woman whose wolf skin was taken from her. She is thus "tamed" and becomes a mother to two sons. Her husband, who hid her old skin away, believed that she was happy in her new domestic role, but as soon as she got the chance, the were-woman stole back her wolfskin, locked her family away and escaped to live the rest of her life in the freedom of the forest. It seems that the old Slavs realized a woman's wild nature is untameable on a deeper level.

Various Slavic rituals called upon the power that wolves symbolized. Some shamans wore wolf skins in order to connect with Veles, ordinary folk wore a wolf tooth as a source of protection and many southern Slavic tribes' childbirth rituals called upon the wolf to protect newborn babies.

In the Polish folk story of "The Wolf and the Devil", a girl is walking home from a market with an apron full of cabbages when she feels something moving around in her apron. She is just about to drop everything, when there is a tug on her skirt – a white wolf with yellow eyes is standing beside her, snarling and baring its sharp, wet teeth. The girl is about to start screaming when a rat jumps out of her apron and the wolf gives chase. When she returns home, her grandma explains that the wolf was her protectant from the devil, symbolized by the rat. We learn that what frightens us may, at times, be a force for good.

The Slavic respect for wolves is reflected in folk art. Wolf teeth may be found in folk art if you know what you are looking for – jagged triangles – an otherworldly source of protection.

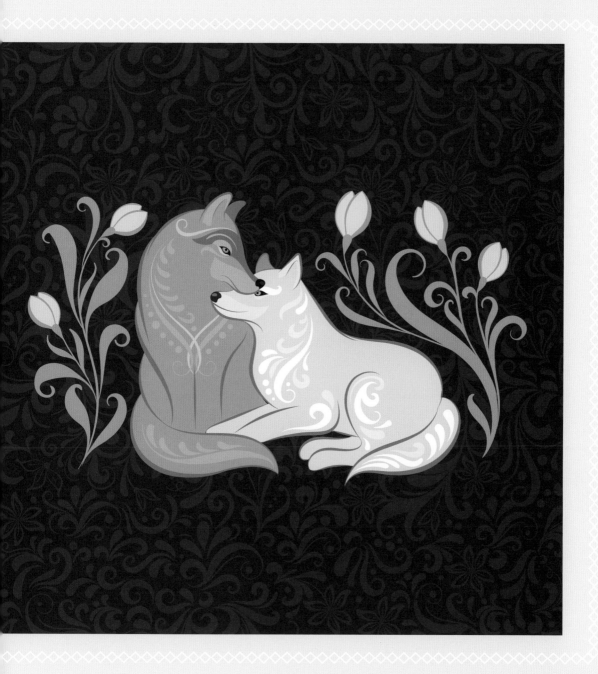

THERAPEUTIC FOLK ARTS FOR WINTER

As the nights draw in and the prospect of going out feels less and less appealing, I suggest we succumb to the winter atmosphere and focus within. A wonderful way to spend a chilly evening is to create something beautiful, either as a gift or to decorate the home before Christmas.

In order to get into any relaxing folk art, we must first prepare our space. A large kitchen table is ideal, if one is available to you. Clear it of any clutter, give it a wipe, then once the environment feels clean and cosy, we can make warm drinks and start the process of creation. It can be done with family or friends, talking softly, connecting gently, but we can also do it alone, connecting with our own deeper selves through the calm, repetitive actions.

STAR OF KURPIE *WYCINANKA*

The Polish folk art of *wycinanki* not only makes a magical Christmas card for someone special, which can be framed and enjoyed for years to come, but is also a highly therapeutic activity, perfect for the dark, cold winter nights. Each region of Poland has its own traditional designs and style of *wycinanki*.

The star is a motif that's repeated in a few different regions of Poland, but this particular technique is most popular in the Kurpie region. Sheep shears were traditionally used to cut out the most intricate of designs and the paper is measured through the means of folding it symmetrically rather than actually measuring

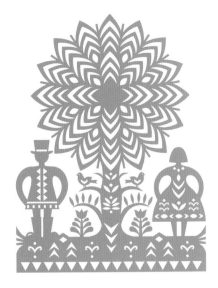

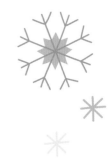

anything. **The brilliant thing about this technique is that it has almost infinite variations and you can make it more intricate with practice. It's a great winter activity to do with children once they can safely use a pair of scissors.**

MAKES 1 DECORATION

A piece of A4 paper
Scissors

1 You need a square, so when we take an A4 piece of paper, we first fold a corner of one of the short sides in to make a triangle. Next, cut off the remaining strip at the end. If you open the triangle, you will now have a square. Fold the triangle up again, then again into another smaller triangle, and again, into an even smaller one. Now, to make a circle, start cutting about 2cm (1in) from the corner of the triangle (the one that forms the centre of the piece of paper) upward in a half moon shape.

2 Open the rounded triangle up just once. Now fold the two outward corners into the middle, so that the edges of the paper meet on the middle line. Then, fold in half once more.

3 Time to start cutting: cut off the top edges, the bottom and go down each side. A popular design in the Kurpie region is the wolf

teeth and *piórka* – feathers. The wolf's teeth are long, sharp, jagged triangles, while the feathers are finer, thinner lines. Leave about 1–2mm between each cut. As a rule, we tend to start with the larger shapes first and get thinner the further down we go.

4 Open up the triangles into the full circle shape.

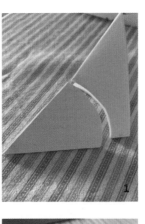

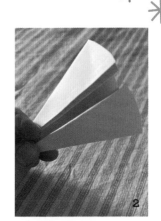

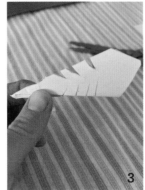

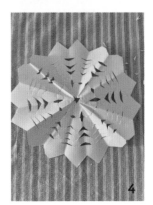

RYE CHAIN for a natural tree and a peaceful afternoon

Most of the decorations on my tree are natural straw-coloured ones that I have bought in Poland, woven by hand into bauble shapes and bought for not much money, usually from the beautifully gnarled hands that wove them. These kinds of decorations make my heart sing, because they have soul. Here and there, you will find a colourful paper decoration that I learned to make at my friend Karolina Merska's workshop.

This chain is a wonderfully simple way to begin working with rye straw, so if you feel intimidated by the beautiful Christmas *pająk* (opposite), I suggest you start here.

Making this rye chain while drinking cups of lemon tea (with some rosehip vodka for immunity – see page 129) is the most pleasant and therapeutic way to spend an afternoon. You could just use the foil and the straw if you want to make a simple version and let go of thinking completely. You could also use pretty beads between the straws or even dried peas in the old way (soak them overnight so that you can thread them). I like to alternate a shiny ball of foil with a coloured fan, because this is the version that I remember so fondly from a childhood tree. You can make the chain longer, but be warned that it's easy to tangle yourself up and then the afternoon becomes less peaceful. If you want to place it all over the tree, it may be an idea to make two or three chains, getting a bit longer with each one. In terms of the fans, any paper that can hold a crease is fine. I like to use origami paper.

MAKES 1 DECORATION

4 x 8cm (1½ x 3¼in) squares
   of coloured paper
16 x 6cm (6½ x 2½in) squares
   of tin foil
1.6–1.8m (64–72in) strong
   thread or string
Large needle
1.5m (60in) rye straw, cut into
   10cm (4in) strips

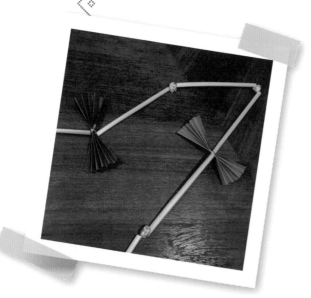

◉ Make the fans first. Lay your squares of paper in front of you and make little creases of about 2mm each – first on one side, then on the other, to create a small concertina.

◉ Make your foil balls, by scrunching them up and rolling them around between your palms.

◉ Thread your needle and make a large knot on the end of the string. Use the needle to poke the thread through the first foil ball. Pull the ball right down to the end.

◉ Now, pull the thread through the first straw and pull it to the end.

◉ Add another ball and another straw.

◉ Then take a concertina and wrap the thread around it in the middle twice to create a fan. Make a double knot to secure it in place, snugly next to the straw. It helps to hold the chain up now, or perhaps hang it up. Pull out the edges of the fan to open it up.

◉ Thread on another piece of straw and repeat until the entire thread is covered in rye straws, paper fans and silver balls, then tie the ends together to create a circle shape.

◉ Finish by combining both ends and trimming the excess string.

RYE STRAW *PAJĄK* CHRISTMAS DECORATIONS

In Poland, Ukraine, Slovenia, Lithuania and Belarus, *pajaki* rye straw chandeliers are used to ward off negativity in the home. They may look incredibly intricate, but they're not difficult to make; it just takes time and patience. My friend Karolina Merska is an expert in the art of *pająki* and has written a book all about it: *Making Mobiles: Create Beautiful Polish Pajaki From Natural Materials*. She has kindly devised a miniature version especially for us that you can hang up in your home or on the tree, as you like. Rye straws are the strongest, but you can use wheat ones too. These days, you can buy them as eco drinking straws on the internet.

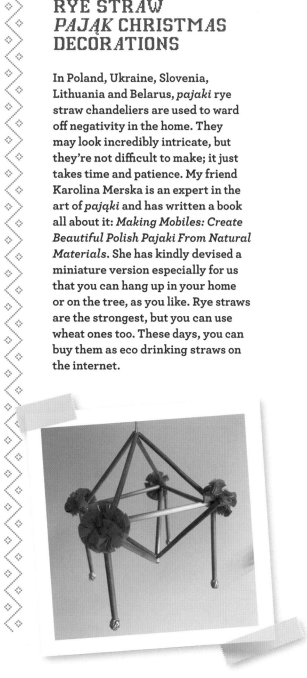

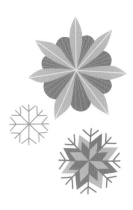

MAKES 1 DECORATION

12 rye straw pieces – 8 x 8cm (3¼in)
    and 4 x 6cm (2½in)
String
Tissue paper in your favourite
    colour
Kitchen foil
Needle/long embroidery needle
Scissors
3cm (1½in) Circle paper puncher
    (or you can cut them out by hand)

1 Using a needle, thread eight of the 8cm (3¼in) rye straws onto 80cm (32in) of the string. Tie a knot at the top.

2 Place on your worktop and twist in the middle twice, as shown in the image, so you have two diamond shapes.

3 Fold one diamond up, then connect at the top with a knot.

4 Tie a piece of string around the middle of one of the sides of the structure.

5 Thread on the next 8cm (3¼in) piece of straw and make a knot at the other end of the straw to secure it to the adjacent side.

6 Starting from where you have just secured the previous straw, thread on another straw and tie it to the next adjacent middle joint, and secure with knot as before.

7 Repeat this process around all the sides with the remaining straws to create a horizontal square within your diamond structure. Trim the string on the knots.

8 Add string on the top to create a hanging loop. Make sure the knot is at the bottom so it's not visible.

9 Cut four circles with 10 layers from your tissue paper using the paper puncher.

10 Insert a needle through the middle of a circle.

11 Make four cuts in the circle.

12 Fold the circle in half and make another eight cuts, four in each quarter.

13 Prepare a square of foil, about 4 x 4cm (1½ x 1½in) in size. Double thread the needle with 10–12cm (4–4½in) of string and wrap the foil around the two ends of the string.

14 Thread through the hole in the centre of your flower and fluff. Double knot and cut off the needle.

15 Repeat steps 10–14 for each of the four flowers.

16 Cut four big squares of foil, about 6cm (2in) in size and four pieces of string, about 15–20cm (6–8in) in length. Tie a knot at one end of each string piece, then wrap a piece of foil around it to create a ball.

17 Hang up the main structure you created in the first eight steps.

18 Thread each piece of string through the remaining 6cm (2½in) rye straw pieces, so that each one has a silver ball on one side. Attach the hanging arms to each corner of the hanging structure.

19 Tie a flower to each corner with two knots. Trim any unwanted string. You can now hang your *pajqk* wherever you want.

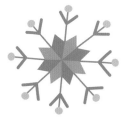

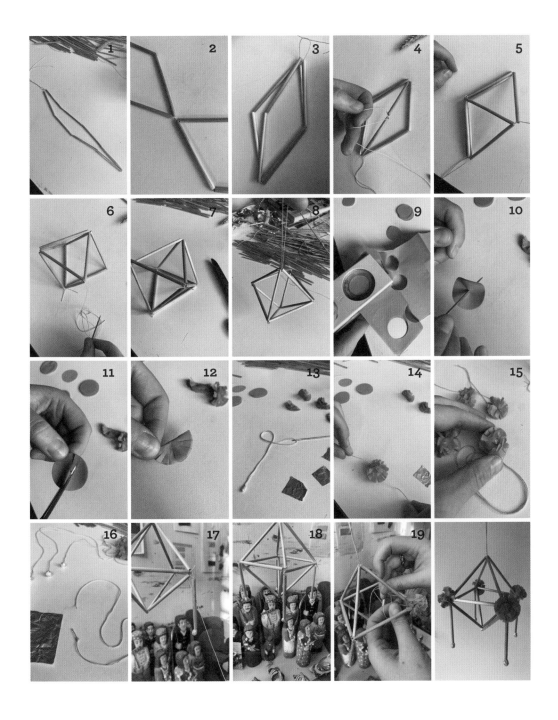

WALNUT CHRISTMAS TREE DECORATIONS
for prosperity

It was a few years ago that my mama had a flashback from her childhood of making these little decorations for the Christmas tree. It harks back to the old days, when apples, walnuts and gingerbread were used to decorate the tree. Even fried dumplings were sometimes used as Christmas tree decorations! (You'll find those in my previous book, *Pierogi*.)

Each member of the family has to make one of these and hang them on the tree themselves in order to have prosperity for the year ahead.

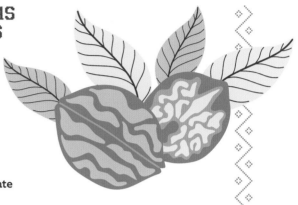

MAKES AS MANY DECORATIONS AS YOU LIKE

Walnuts
Squares of kitchen foil that will fit all the way around a walnut (about 10cm/4in)
A piece of string for each walnut – about 15–20cm (6–8in) in length

◙ Tie the string around the walnut and make a double knot on the nut. Make a loop with the string and tie a knot to keep it in place.

◙ Place the foil, with the less shiny side down, on the table and put the walnut on top, in the middle.

◙ Crumple the foil around the walnut, so that you end up with a shiny ball with the loop sticking out of it.

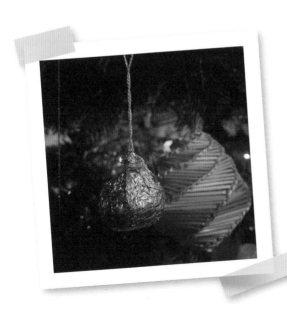

BEETROOT LIP AND CHEEK TINT for a healthy, radiant complexion

Beetroot has been used in the Slavic lands for generations to improve the complexion and give the cheeks and lips a beautiful colour. My daughter discovered this happy by-product of eating beetroot when she was about three years old and paints herself (rather dramatically) every time she eats it. This is a more natural, adult version of the ruddy look.

MAKES 1 X 50ml/2fl oz JAR

1 small beetroot, the size of a walnut
1 tablespoon lemon juice
1 tablespoon unrefined hemp seed
    oil
4 drops rose essential oil
50ml/2fl oz sterilized glass jar
Dark-coloured glass bottle with
    a dropper

◉ Peel and juice your beetroot. If you don't have a juicer, then grate the beetroot and squeeze the juice out through a sieve. You should have about 1 tablespoon of juice.

◉ In your sterilized jar, combine the beetroot juice with the lemon juice. Screw the lid on and shake.

◉ In a bowl, mix the oils thoroughly. Add the mixture to the beetroot jar and shake vigorously again.

◉ Ideally, transfer this to a dark-coloured glass bottle with a dropper, although you can keep it in the jar. Every time you use it, give the bottle a shake

◉ This will keep for about 2 weeks in the refrigerator.

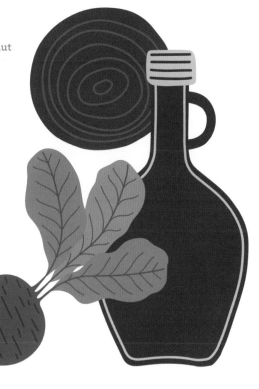

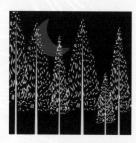

THE MAGIC OF PINE

The first pine Christmas trees of these lands were hung from the ceiling down, decorated with nuts, apples and pretty cookies, then colourful paper decorations in later years. In pre-Christian times, the winter solstice celebrations involved something that symbolized the Tree of Life; often, this was a wheat sheaf, though pine branches were decorated in the Ukraine as part of ancient wedding celebrations. Pine is known to protect, and that was probably their function during those rites.

Pine trees have always been much-loved in the Slavic lands for their warm, supportive energy. It is one of the oldest trees known to man. If oak symbolizes the father, linden the mother and birch the children, pine was seen as the energy of the grandparents. Some still say that pine is the only tree open to human contact, a tree that may help you in times of need. In Slavic folk medicine, pine was known to help coughs and colds and preparing a syrup out of the young pine buds is still practised by some grandmothers to this day.

Most of the ancient Slavic lands used to be covered in pine forests, creating a symbiotic relationship between humans and pines. Some pine forests, where the trees are misshapen and gnarly, have a reputation as a place of dark magic and evil happenings. Other pine forests were deemed sacred, and if anyone cut a tree from one of those, they would be exposed to misfortune. Strict rules were therefore observed in order for the human–nature balance to be maintained.

Pine is used to make the Slavic *banya* (sauna), which, over the years, was a place not only of relaxation, but also of spiritual reflection. In the days when people were trying to hide their pagan rituals, the *banya* was a place where they could safely be performed. The *banya* was said to have its own spirit – *Bannik* – which is why people often make the sign of the cross when they enter. As a result of its protective aura, pine was also used to make wands for magical spells and amulets for those in need of protection. The dead were cremated with pine, and later they were buried in a pine coffin instead.

PINE BATH DECOCTION for a good night's sleep

A decoction is basically an infusion that has been cooked for a while. This helps with getting all the goodness out of certain trees. Since the pine tree (*Pinus sylvestris*) is quite tough, we prepare a decoction to get as much of the oil out as possible. Pine is one of my favourite smells, but I can only get its full effect when the pine needles are warmed by the sun. Then, my whole body immediately relaxes. This bath gives me a similar feeling. You can also drink this decoction – simply take a cup of it and sweeten with honey.

MAKES 1 DECOCTION

30cm (12in) branch of pine
1l/35fl oz/4¼ cups water

◉ Cut the pine branch into 5 or 6 smaller parts with some scissors and place in a large saucepan.

◉ Pour the water over the top and bring to the boil, then cover, turn the heat down a bit and allow to simmer for about 30 minutes. Turn the heat off and allow to cool slightly before using.

◉ Prepare a warm bath, pour the decoction into it and mix in with your hand.

◉ Soak for a minimum of 20 minutes before bed.

PINE AND BEESWAX FURNITURE POLISH for wooden items

The heady smell of pine has the ability to transport us to a wintry pine forest. When I close my eyes and smell pine, I am surrounded by glistening snow, the sun shining onto the wispy pine branches, allowing them to release their magical scent. Once the Christmas tree is gone, I tend to miss that smell, which is why I make this simple furniture polish that works wonders on wood. When using beeswax on my face, I always choose organic, but for a furniture polish, you don't need to spend the extra money.

MAKES 1 JAR

100g/3½oz beeswax
1 tablespoon pine essential oil
2 tablespoons flaxseed oil
150ml/5fl oz sterilized glass jar

◉ Place the beeswax in the jar and place the jar in a saucepan of water over a low heat, making sure that the water comes about halfway up the jar. Allow the water to simmer until the wax melts.

◉ Mix the essential oil with the flaxseed oil in a small bowl.

◉ Once the wax has melted, turn the heat off and add the oil mixture. Stir until thoroughly combined, then leave to cool.

ELDERBERRY BARK INFUSION for winter immunity

In ancient times, trees were believed to be inhabited by deities and, in some East European countries, the belief that trees are a vehicle for souls persists still. Harming trees is therefore strictly forbidden, while using them for health and nutrition is positively encouraged. I learned to do this from a couple in Dolny Śląsk who call themselves the *Chwastożercy* – the weed eaters. They are food anthropologists promoting the old Slavic ways (see acknowledgements) who taught me that, even during the winter months, we can gain health benefits from trees if we learn how to use them in the correct way. One way to do this is by harvesting the bark of certain trees, such as the elderberry, and using it to make tea. The elderberry has a thin brownish bark with a green inner layer. In the olden days, people would always thank the elder as they took what they needed for their health purposes.

SERVES 2-4

40–50cm (16–20in) branch
    of elderberry
Sharp knife, or a vegetable peeler
Hot water from a pre-boiled kettle
Sterilized glass jar or ziplock bag

◙ Wash the elderberry twig, then allow it to dry. The very same day, use a sharp knife or a vegetable peeler to shave the bark off the twig.

◙ Leave the shavings to dry for 2-3 days in a well-ventilated place away from the sun.

◙ Crush the shavings in a pestle and mortar or a food processor. Store these shavings in your sterilized (and thoroughly dried) jar or ziplock bag. They will keep for up to 6 months.

◙ Place 1 heaped teaspoon of the bark in a mug and pour over hot water. Cover and allow to infuse for about 20 minutes, then strain and drink. You could pour this into a thermos flask to keep warm and drink throughout the day too.

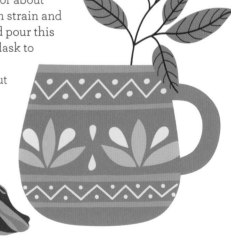

WILLOW BARK INFUSION for headaches

The willow's (*Salix*) salicin is said to be the inspiration for aspirin, so you can imagine the strong compounds that it must contain. The ancient Slavs used its bark to treat headaches and coughs and it was even said to help with a fever. Swallowing a pussy willow, on the other hand, was said to ensure prosperity for the whole year. A word of caution: as a child, I put a pussy willow up my nose (I liked its smell so much) and nearly ended up in hospital, so they should be kept out of reach of young children.

The bark of a tree is like its skin – a vital protective layer. We do not want to remove a lot of the tree's bark, as it may then be vulnerable to insect infestation. The best way to take bark for our purposes is to simply prune a branch off the tree without damaging its central trunk.

SERVES 2-4

40–50cm (16–20in) branch
  of willow
Sharp knife, or a vegetable peeler
Hot water from a pre-boiled kettle
Sterilized glass jar or ziplock bag

◉ Wash the willow twig, then allow it to dry. The very same day, use a sharp knife or a vegetable peeler to shave the bark off the twig.

◉ Leave the shavings to dry for 2–3 days in a well-ventilated place away from the sun.

◉ Crush the shavings in a pestle and mortar or a food processor. Store these shavings in your sterilized (and fully dried) jar or ziplock bag. They will keep for up to 6 months.

◉ Place 1 heaped teaspoon of the bark in a mug and pour over hot water. Cover and allow to infuse for about 20 minutes, then strain and drink. You could pour this into a thermos flask to keep warm and drink throughout the day too.

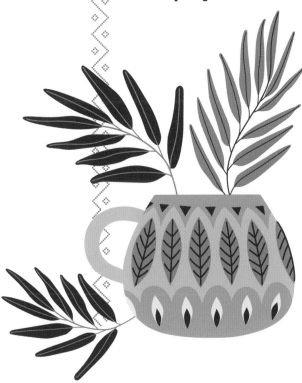

HEMP SEED SOUP for no more sore throats

It is estimated that the Slavs have used hemp since 1400 BCE to make ropes, clothing and food. In certain areas of Poland, there used to be a soup made from hemp milk and *kasza*, called *siemieniotka*, which was reputed to protect you from a sore throat for the entire coming year if eaten on Christmas Eve. I imagine eating it on New Year's Eve could work too! It's a soup that's known in a few of the other Slavic countries too, in various guises.

SERVES 4

100g/3½oz roasted buckwheat (*kasza*)
2 tablespoons butter
1 tablespoon cold-pressed
    rapeseed/canola oil
1 onion, finely chopped
1 carrot, grated
300g/10½oz hulled hemp seeds
2l/70fl oz/8½ cups water
1 tablespoon flour
3 tablespoons sour cream
1 teaspoon sugar
1 tablespoon lemon juice
Salt and black and white pepper,
    to taste

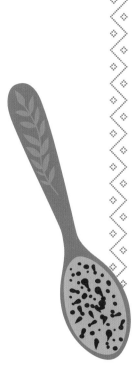

◉ Rinse the buckwheat and place in a saucepan with about 2cm (¾in) of water and a pinch of salt. Cover and bring to the boil, then turn the heat down and simmer for 10–15 minutes until all the water is absorbed. Cover the pan with a dish towel and another thicker layer, and place somewhere warm to steam for 30–40 minutes.

◉ Meanwhile, melt 1 tablespoon of the butter in a pan over a medium heat, then add the rapeseed oil and onion. Sauté for about 5 minutes until softened. Add the grated carrot and sauté for a further 10 minutes, stirring regularly. Add the hemp seeds and cook for another minute.

◉ Cover with the water and bring to the boil. Turn the heat down and simmer for 30 minutes. Allow to cool before transfering to a blender and blending until smooth.

◉ Pour a ladleful of the soup into a bowl and add the flour. Mix well to combine – it shouldn't have lumps.

◉ Pour the soup back into the pan and bring to the boil. Turn the heat down and stir for 10 minutes to thicken.

◉ Spoon the sour cream into a bowl and add a tablespoon of soup, then mix well. Repeat with 3 more tablespoons, then stir the mixture back into the pan. Taste and season the soup with the sugar, lemon juice, salt and pepper, then ladle into bowls.

◉ Add 1 tablespoon of butter to the kasza pan and fluff up the kasza before serving on top of the soup.

HONEY AND HEMP SELF-CARE SALVE
for healing the skin

While there is beauty both to winter and to Baba Yaga, we don't necessarily want to look like her before our time. During the winter, we spend so much time indoors that the heating dries out our skin while the elements batter it outdoors. This self-care salve is the answer – it's perfect as a lip balm, eye cream, hand salve or for any rough patches that may show up at this time of year.

Honey is a part of life in many of the Slavic countries. Even the first chronicler of Poland, Gallus Anonymous, mentions it in his writings from the 12th century. Honey has medicinal properties, but, of course, this is all dependent on the quality of the honey, on the way it's produced and the like. Therefore, we need to use the best-quality honey we can get.

Then there's hemp (*Cannabis sativa*) – one of those miracle plants that offers so many gifts to use yet has become demonized because of its close relative marijuana. However, I believe that we are coming back to understanding its great versatility and sustainability, so perhaps it will play a lead role in our wellbeing once more in the future.

MAKES 1 X 150ml/5fl oz JAR

10g/¼oz organic unprocessed beeswax
150ml/5fl oz/⅔ cup unrefined hemp seed oil
1 teaspoon good-quality honey
150ml/5fl oz sterilized glass jar

◉ Place the beeswax in the jar and melt in a saucepan of water over a low heat, making sure that the water comes about halfway up the jar.

◉ Add the oil and stir regularly so that the two combine thoroughly (I like to use the back of a small wooden spoon for this). When combined, stir in the honey, thoroughly mixing it in.

◉ Turn the heat off and wipe the sides of your jar while still warm. Once the water starts to cool a little, you can remove the jar, screw the lid on and allow the salve to cool to room temperature.

◉ This healing salve will keep for at least 3 months at room temperature.

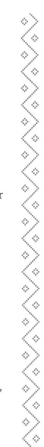

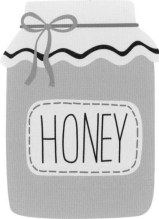

HONEY

BABA YAGA THE CRONE

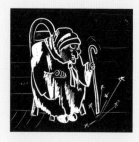

Baba Yaga the crone is known by all Slavs as the scary witch who lives in a gnarly pine forest, in a hut standing on chicken legs. Known by many names, including the Ancient Goddess of Old Bones and the White Lady of Death and Rebirth, she has sadly turned into a two-dimensional figure in our youth-obsessed modern world. How shallow we have become that the ancient Slavic Goddess of Death and Rebirth has become an ugly, old woman with the sole purpose of frightening little children. Baba Yaga's true story is as rich and enticing as she is.

In old folk stories, Baba Yaga often helped people in difficult situations, as long as they were smart and brave. While she disliked stupidity and cowardice, she wasn't a cruel being. In fact, she was incredibly useful. In the Polish story "The Dragon", she betrays her grandson, the tricky dragon, because she is impressed by the courage and intelligence of a young man who escaped from the army. She allows him to listen to her conversation with the dragon, so he can overhear the answers to the dragon's riddle. In a Russian folk tale, "The Feather of Finist the Falcon", three Baba Yagas give the hero advice and magical gifts to help him on his journey. In some Slavic folk tales, Baba Yaga presided over the last sheaf of harvested grain; whoever bound that grain would be blessed with a child in the coming spring.

We fear Baba Yaga because she represents the frightening unknown, death and shadows. Meeting her forces us to go deep within ourselves, to the place where we have hidden away all the things we don't like to look at, our own shadow.

Despite our society's pushing away of Baba Yaga, the crone lives on. She manifests herself in wise, old women, such as the whisperers of Poland. These crones whisper incantations to help whoever comes to them. Despite their witchy ways, these women are usually very religious and maintain that God uses them to heal. Rather like my own grandmother, Babcia Ziuta, who, despite going to church at 6am every single day, would use the old way now and again when a family member needed help. I was told that she would take them into a separate room, whisper unknown words, lick their eyelids, then spit in every corner of the room.

Summer never lasts for ever and change is certain for all of us. It is up to us to uncover and accept the beauty in every age. In the winter of our lives, we should hopefully know the wisdom of Baba Yaga and be grateful for her gifts.

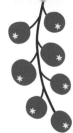

ROWANBERRY INFUSION to keep the north wind and illnesses at bay

The bright-red rowanberry (*Sorbus aucuparia*) popping against a sea of white is one of the quintessential symbols of winter. Eaten uncooked, the berries could give you a bad stomach, yet we only need to prepare them in the simplest of ways to benefit from their goodness. Rowanberries are rich in vitamin C, which will give you a much-need immunity boost at this time of year. They're also known to help the kidneys, so you could use them for urinary tract health, if needed. We want to collect rowanberries that are fully ripe, so look for a bright red colour, rather than an orange.

To dry:

Spread the rowanberries out on a baking sheet lined with greaseproof/wax paper. Place in the oven at 60°C/140°F for 30 minutes, then turn the oven down to 50°C/120°F for an hour. Turn the oven off and leave them in there for a further hour or so. Once cool, keep the rowanberries in an airtight container for up to 3 months.

SERVES 1

1 teaspoon dried rowanberries
250ml/9fl oz/1 cup hot water from a pre-boiled kettle
1 teaspoon good-quality honey
Thermos flask

◉ Place the dried rowanberries in a thermos flask and cover with the hot (but not boiling) water.

◉ Close the flask and allow to infuse for 2–3 hours, then strain out the berries, add the honey and pour the infusion back into the flask. Drink throughout the day. You could also pour hot water over the rowanberries in a mug, cover it with a saucer and drink after 20 minutes.

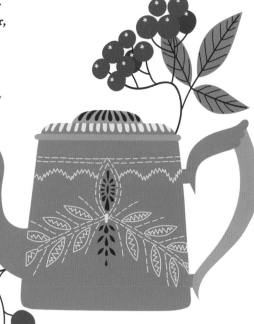

THE NORTH WIND
(A Polish story)

There once lived a cold-hearted peasant woman who had a daughter named Kasieńka and a stepdaughter named Inek. In the woman's eyes, Kasieńka could do no wrong, whereas poor Inek had a very hard time. She was helpful and kind, yet her stepmother could not bear the sight of her.

"Send Inek away", she begged her husband daily. "Send her away into the fields, and if the *polewiki* don't get her, the North Wind will."

The father was a weak-willed man, afraid to be alone, and knew that he'd married a dark witch. One day he unexpectedly succumbed to his wife's demands. He put Inek in a sled and drove her out into the cold, bare fields. He kissed her goodbye and quickly drove back, not daring to look back.

Deserted and alone, Inek sat under a rowan tree on the edge of a forest and wept silently. After a time,

tiredness washed over her. She was starting to feel ready to let go of her miserable life on earth, when she heard a strange sound. It was the North Wind running through the forest, cracking his fingers and whistling an otherworldy tune. Eventually, he reached the rowan tree and landed beside her.

"Don't you know who I am?", his voice whistled and blew icy air in her direction. "I am the North Wind, the King of Winter, who turns the rivers to ice and ground to stone. I am Cold and Death and I bring death to you too, little one."

"Greetings to you, Mighty King," said Inek, "so you have come to chill to my bones."

The North Wind considered for a moment, as if recognizing something in the girl, then he cocked his head to one side and said:

"Are you warm, Maiden?"

"I'm quite warm, my lord", replied Inek, her lips turning blue.

The King of Winter bent over her and the cracking sound grew loud, the air colder still. "Are you warm now, my lovely child?"

Inek whispered as bravely as she could: "I'm quite toasty, thank you, my lord."

The North Wind tested her one last time. He cracked his fingers and howled and blew louder and frostier than ever. "Are you still warm now, little dove?"

Inek could barely gasp. She summoned all her remaining strength and said: "Oh, yes, I'm still warm, so kind of you to ask."

The North Wind was so impressed by the girl's courtesy and uncomplaining ways, that he took pity on her. He wrapped her in furs and called for his sled. Six silvery horses appeared from the blizzard, drawing an icy white sled. The King of Winter promptly took the girl to his castle, where he gave her gifts of a rich robe embroidered in silver and gold and a chest full of sparkling jewels. He told her to warm herself by the fire and then he would take her home.

Meanwhile, at home, the wicked stepmother was happily humming to herself while preparing pancakes for Inek's funeral feast. She said to her long-suffering husband: "Old fool, you had better go and find her body and bring it home."

The sad, old man nodded but just as he was getting ready to go, the dog began to bark.

"Your daughter shall live to be your delight and her daughter will die this very night", it said in a human voice.

The woman kicked the dog and shouted: "I conjured the power of speech for you to talk such rubbish!" But quickly she changed her tune and gave the dog a pancake. "You must now say: 'Her daughter will have much silver and gold, his daughter is frozen dead and cold.'" The dog ate the pancake and wagged his tail happily, then said: "His daughter shall wear a crown on her head, her daughter will

die unwed." When giving him more pancakes didn't work, the woman beat the dog to try and make it say what she wanted, but to no avail.

Suddenly, the door creaked open and there was Inek, looking like an otherworldly mirage, glittering in silver and gold. For a moment, even the witch's eyes were dazzled.

"Where did you get those riches?!" she snapped.

"The North Wind gave them to me", Inek replied.

The woman called to her husband: "Old fool, take the horses at once and leave my daughter in the exact spot you left yours. She must get her dues."

The old man did as he was told and left Kasieńka in the exact same spot he'd left Inek, then returned home, as he had done before.

When the North Wind came to Kasieńka, he asked her: "Are you warm, Maiden?"

"What?" she replied angrily "Are you blind as well as ugly? I'm freezing! It's winter and my stupid mother has sent me out into a blizzard!"

This angered the North Wind, and he froze her on the spot.

At home, the woman grew impatient and snapped at her husband: "Why are you just standing there? Her chest is probably too big to carry, go out and help her."

The little dog barked: "Your daughter is frozen stiff and cold."

"Wicked beast!" screamed the woman "I'll give you a pancake if you just say ..."

But she didn't have time to finish her sentence, for the door blew open and there stood the North Wind:

"Mother, are you warm ...?"

A FINAL NOTE

I believe that we are all on a journey of growth and development through the challenges that we face. Life isn't always easy, yet what I've learned through my own experiences is that it needn't be complicated, chaotic or confusing either. Beauty, magic, nourishment, wisdom and healing are all around us, and through simple kitchen alchemy they can be ours for the taking.

I hope that this book has already helped you align with the rhythms of nature in the way practised by Slavic grandmothers and folk practitioners for generations. It contains all the recipes that work for me – the ones that help me feel grounded, connected, and confident in my own abilities, in my body and in Mother Nature. The ones that bring me comfort and joy.

I also hope that you have added your own recipes and notes to it, that you have written in the margins, attached cut-outs from magazines and scribbled handy sketches to make this book unique to you – and you will continue to do so as the seasons change and the years go by. Sometimes we underestimate all that we already know and risk losing those important little bits of wisdom to time. I implore you to continue to write it all down here as a gift to future generations.

My final hope is that reading this book has done the same for you as writing it did for me: that it has been a gentle reminder of the magical nature of our existence here on this planet, where we already have everything that we need and it's just a matter of finding it. As my youngest daughter says every day, no matter what we are about to do, "We are going on an adventure."

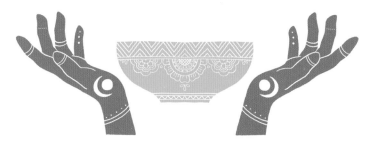

ACKNOWLEGEMENTS

This book was born in a conversation with Fiona Robertson at Watkins. Thank you Fiona for your openness and belief in this project. Thank you also to my agent Isabel Atherton at Creative Authors for the unfaltering enthusiasm and belief in me.

A huge thank you to the team who made it all come alive - Brittany Willis, Sophie Elletson, Ella Chappell and Karen Smith; illustrator Kira Konoshenko and front cover designer Alice Coleman. I am so grateful for all your work on this project.

To the experts and authors who contributed to this book: cultural anthropologist and folk craft practitioner Karolina Merska; foraging expert Chwastozercy (*Ancient Slow Food*, see page 202); Slavic witchcraft expert Natasha Helvin; and food anthropologist Darra Goldstein.

To all the people who have supported and inspired me along the way - a huge thank you to Julia Jendrych for the bag of herbal magazines and books that magically appeared on my doorstep in Poland, my aunt Wiesia for the inspiration she gave me in Ciechocinek, Marta Bagińska for passing on her wisdom and my physio, Magda, for all the informative conversations (and the brilliant massages, of course).

To my family for their constant love and support - without which I wouldn't be able to do anything! My mother, Teresa, who is with me on every book journey. My father, Kajetan, and my brother, Robert, who are supportive of all my endeavours. My in-laws, Patricia and Ovidio, who are on hand to help whenever I need them. And finally, a massive thank you to my partner, Yasin, for his practical and emotional support every day, and our girls, Delfina and Kazimira, for their existence in our lives.

ABOUT THE AUTHOR

Zuza Zak is a Polish author and cook with an interest in using storytelling to delve into another cuisine and, through it, into another culture. She learned the arts of cooking and foraging from an early age from her beloved Babcias. Zuza is now passing on her culinary love to her daughters through storytelling and fun learning. Her aim is to inspire the world to cook and eat more food from Eastern Europe

Zuza's previous books include *Polska, Amber & Rye* and *Pierogi*. You can also see Zuza across Europe and the Middle East presenting Polish food in *Food Network Finds: Poland.*

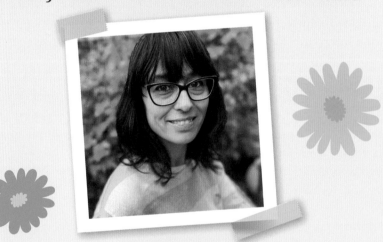

ABOUT THE ILLUSTRATOR

Kira Konoshenko is a Ukrainian illustrator. She graduated from the Lviv Academy of Arts. For a long time, she was engaged in the manufacture of souvenirs from glass and ceramics. When the coronavirus pandemic began, and the tourist industry stalled, she began to draw and illustrate.

After the war began in Ukraine. she decided to leave the country with her nine-year-old daughter. They lived for some time in Poland, before moving in with a very nice family in England. They currently live in Ickleton, Cambridgeshire.

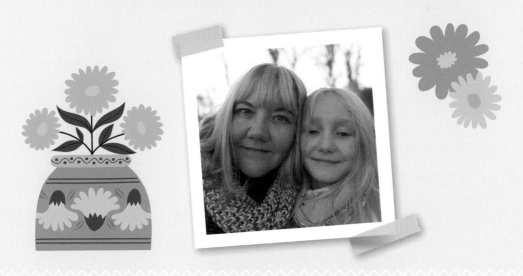

FURTHER RESOURCES

BOOKS

Asala, Joanne (ed), *Polish Folklore and Myth*, Penfield Books, McFarland & Company Inc, 2013

Bane, T, *Encyclopedia of Fairies in World Folklore and Mythology*, McFarland & Company, 2013

Bobrowski J and Wrona, M, *Mitologia Słowiańska*, Bosz Publishing House, 2017

Chwastozercy, *Ancient Slow Food*, chwastozercy.gumroad.com, online

Goldstein, D, *Beyond the North Wind: Russia in Recipes and Lore*, Ten Speed Press, 2020

Helvin N, *Slavic Witchcraft: Old World Conjuring Spells and Folklore*, 2019

Horodowicz-Knabb, S, *Polish Herbs, Flowers and Folk Medicine*, Hippocrene Books, 2020

Hoffman, D, *Holistic herbal: A Safe and Practical Guide to Making and Using Herbal Medicines*, Harper Collins, 1990

Pinkola Estés, C, *Women Who Run With the Wolves*, Mass Market Paperback, 1996

Merska, K, *Making Mobiles: Create Beautiful Polish Pajaki From Natural Materials*, Pavilion Books, 2021

Moszyński, K, *Kultura Ludowa Słowian: Kultura Duchowa*, Polska Akademia Umiejętności, 1934

Nisbet Bain, R (ed), *Cossack Fairy Tales and Folk-Tales*, George Harrap, 1916 (originally published 1894)

Laprus, J, *Słowiańskie Boginki Ziół*, Świat Książki, 2021

Petrovitch, W M, *Hero Tales and Legends of the Serbians*, George G Harrap & Co. Ltd, Ebook, The Project Gutenberg, 1914

Udziela M, *Medycyna i przesądy lecznicze ludu polskiego: przyczynek do etnografii polskiej*, skł. gł. w księgarni M. Arcta, Warszawa, 1891

Zawistowska, Z, *Przetwory Domowe, dawne i nowe*, Instytut Wydawniczy Związków Zawodowych, Warszawa, 1990

PUBLICATIONS

Sr Kaczmarczyk-Sedlak I, Prof Cioołkowski A, Leczenie Ziołami. Część 2, Gazeta Wyborcza, Warszawa, 2018

Torabian G, Valtchev P, Adil Q, Dehghani F, *Anti-influenza activity of elderberry (Sambucus nigra)*, Journal of Functional Foods, Elsevier, March 201

USEFUL INTERNET SITES

WorldofTales.com

Sławosław.pl

blog.slowianskibestiariusz.pl/

www.odkrywamyzakryte.com

kulturaludowa.pl/artykuly/polska-wycinanka-ludowa/

INDEX

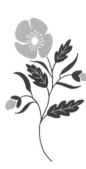